GOOD NEWS FOR ARTHRITIS SUFFERERS!

Revealing how prostaglandins—biochemicals that our bodies produce—either accentuate or relieve arthritis, Dr. James Scala presents proven strategies for making pain-relieving food choices. He provides a complete and delicious 10-day menu plan that includes a delightful collection of irresistible recipes to help you maintain the variety essential to healthy eating. In addition, he gives detailed advice on healthful supplements, along with diet tips and hints for quick pain relief and guidelines for maintaining long-term benefits.

THE ARTHRITIS RELIEF DIET

DR. JAMES SCALA has been involved in nutrition and health research for over twenty years. After completing undergraduate work at Columbia, Dr. Scala received his Ph.D. in biochemistry from Cornell University in 1964. He has taught nutrition at various universities and medical schools in the United States and abroad. His ability to discuss complex nutrition-related health issues in an understandable way makes him a frequent guest on radio and television talk shows.

THE ARTHRITIS RELIEF DIET

by
Dr. James Scala

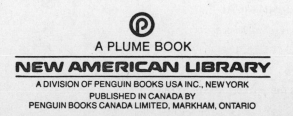

A PLUME BOOK

NEW AMERICAN LIBRARY

A DIVISION OF PENGUIN BOOKS USA INC., NEW YORK
PUBLISHED IN CANADA BY
PENGUIN BOOKS CANADA LIMITED, MARKHAM, ONTARIO

Note to the Reader

The ideas, procedures, and suggestions contained in this book are not intended as a substitute for consulting with your physician. All matters regarding your health require medical supervision.

NAL BOOKS ARE AVAILABLE AT QUANTITY DISCOUNTS WHEN USED TO PROMOTE PRODUCTS OR SERVICES. FOR INFORMATION PLEASE WRITE TO PREMIUM MARKETING DIVISION, NEW AMERICAN LIBRARY, 1633 BROADWAY, NEW YORK, NEW YORK 10019.

The Arthritis Relief Diet previously appeared in an NAL BOOKS edition published by New American Library and simultaneously in Canada by The New American Library of Canada Limited (now Penguin Books Canada Limited).

PLUME TRADEMARK REG. U.S. PAT. OFF. AND FOREIGN COUNTRIES
REGISTERED TRADEMARK—MARCA REGISTRADA
HECHO EN BRATTLEBORO, VT., U.S.A.

SIGNET, SIGNET CLASSIC, MENTOR, ONYX, PLUME, MERIDIAN and NAL BOOKS are published *in the United States* by New American Library, a division of Penguin Books USA Inc., 1633 Broadway, New York, New York 10019, *in Canada* by Penguin Books Canada Limited, 2801 John Street, Markham, Ontario L3R 1B4

Library of Congress Cataloging-in-Publication Data

Scala, James, 1934–
   The arthritis relief diet.

   1. Arthritis—Diet therapy.   3. Arthritis—
Nutritional aspects   I. Title.   [DNLM: 1. Arthritis—
diet therapy—popular works.   2. Cookery.
WE 344 S281a]
RC933.S27   1987   616.7′220654   87-1732
ISBN 0-453-00549-7
ISBN 0-452-26476-6 (pbk)

Designed by Leonard Telesca

First Printing, March, 1989

     6   7   8   9   10   11

PRINTED IN THE UNITED STATES OF AMERICA

To Nancy and our children
Jim, Scott, Greg, Nancy, Kim, Joan, and Juliana

"The summit should always be second to the way you make the climb."

—Ed Hixon, M.D.
North Face of Mt. Everest, 1983

ACKNOWLEDGMENTS

To all of the people who have followed this diet, I express my deepest gratitude. They made this book possible and helped me to learn.

My wife, Nancy, deserves special recognition for typing the manuscript many times over. But Nancy did more; she spoke to people on the diet, helped them, and made it better. She talked with scientists and helped me to sharpen the concepts.

To Kim, many thanks for her help in indexing and checking spelling.

Chris Hollis deserves special thanks for her support, understanding, and help in separating my two worlds.

Carole Hall and Al Zuckerman deserve a special place: Al for getting behind the concept; Carole for her soft-spoken support and encouragement. I will always be grateful.

Contents

V. Getting It All Together: People Helping People

Preface

As a boy I remember my mother being troubled by "rheumatism." When I got older I realized she had a mild case of rheumatoid arthritis. I was distressed about the pain and discomfort it caused her.

My career in nutrition took me into extensive public speaking. Someone in every audience asked what could be done through diet to relieve arthritis. Because I realized just how debilitating and painful a disease it is and how little is known, I began a quest to find a dietary approach for its management.

I surveyed folk remedies because they usually have a scientific foundation. I reviewed the Chinese approach through vegetarian diets. I collected anecdotal information on alfalfa. I followed fasting experiments. They all led me to believe there was even more that diet could do.

During this time, much scientific research was being devoted to the prostaglandins, their metabolism, and EPA. While reading a paper by the Japanese group at Chiba Medical School, I realized that a dietary approach for arthritis was in the dietary management of the prostaglandins. Louis Pasteur said, "Chance favors the mind that is prepared," and I was certainly prepared. Dietary management of the prostaglandins required a carefully planned diet that could be supplemented with EPA for nutritional insurance. So I designed such a diet.

I gave a very abbreviated diet plan to my mother. I described it to people from the podium when I spoke. Then I wrote a shortened version of *Do's* and *Don'ts* for people who wrote to me.

As I write, many people have tried the diet. It works!

I have received many letters, telling about its effectiveness. On speaking engagements, even on a radio phone-in show, people tell me how well it works. The glow in their eyes is worth a million words.

This book is much more complete than the original two-page list of *Do's* and *Don'ts*. I have included all of the "hindsight," as much of the science as is reasonable, and all the folk remedies that work. Most important, I have included the experience of real people.

I believe that every person has something to give his or her fellow shipmates on this beautiful spaceship we call Earth. I want this book to help people with arthritis regain control of their health and return quality to their lives. For me, nothing could be more gratifying.

James Scala

PART I

The Concept: The Right Food Can Help You Feel Better

CHAPTER

1 Your Personal Commitment

Arthritis relief is within *your* power. All you have to do is make a personal commitment to follow the diet revealed in this book.

As the days and weeks pass it will cease to be a diet; indeed, it will become habit and you will wonder how you got along before.

THE PROMISE OF PAIN RELIEF

Hundreds of people have already made this diet commitment. Each one has experienced some relief. The following letter from Ohio is typical of the joyous responses I've received.

Dear Dr. Scala,

A miracle has come into my life. Prior to your diet I had days I could not walk. My hands were double in size. I had severe pain in my entire body. I could not lay down and sleep. My husband had to help me dress and comb my hair. I was taking medicine for pain; not much results. I was diagnosed as having rheumatoid arthritis. Your diet came in the mail at this time. I got on it immediately. I have been very faithful to it and the supplements with great results.

I went back to the doctor yesterday. I was feeling good with only pain in the morning. My muscles were becoming strong again. The doctor was in total shock when he saw me. He said he expected me to be much worse and in severe pain and not really able to walk well. I told him about my diet and he said it was working for sure and not to stop. I have only been on the diet for 14 days.

Dramatic results come quickly once you make your diet commitment, even though some pain and stiffness may still persist.

My diet works in exciting ways. It isn't actually a miracle; it just feels like one! Once you've got arthritis it's here to stay. But your pain can be relieved.

DIET MAKES A DIFFERENCE

"Let food be thy medicine," said Hippocrates around 400 B.C.

Dietary help for the chronically ill is not new. Examples are all around us, including diabetics, kidney patients, and wheelchair-confined paraplegics to name an obvious few. Chronic obesity or chronic underweight are examples so common we never think about them as illnesses.

Indeed, improving one's health through diet isn't confined to ill people. Athletes do it every day. Runners, mountain climbers, skiers, ballerinas, and swimmers are only a few that I have personally advised. And there are as many others as there are sports. Dietary support is probably as old as competition itself.

Some "experts" claim arthritis is different. But they are being proven wrong. Diet *can* help.

THE RIGHT FOOD REDUCES INFLAMMATION

Arthritis is a collection of over 100 diseases affecting one or more joints and in some varieties the major organs. The word *arthritis* literally means inflammation of the joint. "Arth" is taken from the Greek meaning joint and "itis" meaning inflammation or infection.

For most people, the diagnosis of arthritis may have involved many physician visits, lab tests, and examinations. The diagnosis commonly pinpoints one of three arthritic conditions. Each of them can be helped by the diet you are about to begin.

1. *Rheumatoid arthritis* is an inflammatory disease of the tissues inside the joint. It is the most common form of arthritis and is the form my diet is directed toward most specifically. Swollen knees and twisted hands is the image most people have of rheumatoid arthritis. Rheumatoid is the most crippling and painful form of arthritis, but only one of six who get the disease develops deformities—most lead fairly normal lives, albeit with discomfort. With this diet, even that discomfort can be reduced.

2. *Osteoarthritis* is a degenerative disease affecting the bones themselves as the cartilage that covers the movable bones breaks down. Diet will help reduce the inflammation that often accompanies this condition. The weight-control aspect of my diet is important for relieving this form of arthritis.

3. *Gout* is a metabolic disorder, probably hereditary, which leads to the accumulation of uric acid crystals in the joints, especially of the foot, big toe, thumb, and earlobe. Drugs and diet can control gout. The diet in this book is especially helpful.

4. *Other diseases* in which inflammation is a problem can benefit from this diet. These include the scaling of psoriasis,

inflammation in lupus erythematosus, asthma flare-ups, and even migraine headache.

NUTRIENT BALANCE FIGHTS INFLAMMATION

Maybe you're not suffering from a noticeable vitamin or mineral deficiency, but you are likely to be getting less than what is recommended.

How do I know? Studies show that people with arthritis often have less than the recommended daily allowance (RDA) of a number of vitamins and minerals. These include vitamins A and C, one or two B vitamins, the minerals calcium, zinc, copper, iron, and selenium.

These dietary shortfalls are typical of people who don't eat enough total food in sufficient variety. This is not at all surprising. Many people don't get adequate variety, and it is difficult to prepare the variety of foods which will insure that adequate nutrients are obtained when you've got inflammation and the accompanying pain. How does my diet eliminate this shortfall? The diet is well balanced and teaches you to purchase a little nutrition insurance as food supplements, that's how!

Supplementation is an easy way of insuring that the nutrients are always in adequate supply. Any modest excess will be nutrition insurance. A few examples might help.

In my travels I meet arthritis sufferers who simply go on a program of nutritional supplementation and feel much better. They swear that just adding vitamins and minerals to their diet has cured their disease. They are surprised when I tell them it hasn't cured it, but the supplements have elevated their general health so their body can deal with the problem more effectively. My diet will show you how to start supplementing to the RDA now; it will build your nutritional foundation and help your diet work wonders.

DIETARY FIBER FIGHTS INFLAMMATION

One more natural food substance is going to help your diet work: fiber, the nondigestible plant material we call roughage. The old saying, "An apple a day keeps the doctor away" was a way of teaching that fiber and the regularity it produces are essential for good health. It is absolutely vital for arthritics.

Think of dietary fiber as a special brush. A brush that not only sweeps things along, but a brush that also selectively binds materials to its bristles. These two qualities work together and their effects are synergistic. They produce unexpected results. Our objective is to make sure we get enough dietary fiber to sweep things along and the correct types of fiber to remove selectively all those things we don't need.

SHAKE OFF ARTHRITIC PAIN

In the next few chapters I'll explore inflammation more deeply and show you how to loosen its grip on your body.

You'll learn why inflammation is moderated by diet.

You'll see why you should take out a nutrition insurance policy in the form of sensible supplementation and added fiber.

I want you to be so successful on this plan that it will become a way of life. You will exchange old eating habits for new ones. You will learn to identify sensitive foods that cause inflammation and to satisfy all your basic nutritional needs.

The Arthritis Relief Diet is going to help put you back in control of your health.

CHAPTER

2 The Push-Pull of Inflammation

Even though arthritis is a complex of about 100 diseases, most of them have one common factor: inflammation.

Flare-ups are the periods of inflammation and pain that seem to come to the arthritis sufferer from nowhere. Research has shown that flare-ups are associated with changes in the barometric pressure, which explains why people who have arthritis can predict weather changes. Flare-ups often follow periods of mental stress and they accompany physical stress. Most important for our purposes, flare-ups can be caused by foods. The Arthritis Relief Diet works because it:

- Reduces the things in your diet that cause flare-ups,
- Increases the things in your diet that reduce flare-ups

This chapter will explain the scientific connection between food and flare-ups.

A MARVELOUS MACHINE BREAKS DOWN

Your body is the most marvelous living machine ever designed, and each joint is a masterpiece of the Creator's bioengineering. Joints can bear a tremendous amount of weight—up to 400 pounds of pressure on knees, hips, and ankles with each step, yet you can glide smoothly across the dance floor.

Healthy joints have a firm rubbery material called cartilage to cover the bone and act as a shock absorber to cushion the weight of a step or the pressure of a pull. Cartilage also lubricates the bones to keep the ends from grinding against each other. The joint is then held together by ligaments and tendons. Tendons are strong, flexible, biological cables that attach the muscles to the bones and allow movement in various directions. The bone ends, cartilage, ligaments, and tendons are enclosed by a membrane—the synovial membrane. It produces synovial fluid, nature's oil to lubricate the joint so it can move smoothly and easily.

In arthritic joints a breakdown occurs in the tissues that normally allow freedom of movement; they become inflamed and they hurt.

In rheumatoid arthritis the synovial membrane becomes inflamed, which limits normal activity. It can turn even the simplest task into an ordeal. As the joint continues to be inflamed, the body attempts to protect itself and the synovial membrane begins growing; if increased growth continues long enough, the synovial membrane can become so overgrown and convoluted that the joint will become totally deformed and, for most practical purposes, useless. In arthritic inflammation, the body is its own worst enemy.

THE ONSET OF INFLAMMATION

Our bodies function as chemical processing plants. We each consist of trillions of cells. Each cell can perform thousands of biochemical reactions. Among those reactions, it makes three biochemicals that scientists named prostaglandins.

Two of the three prostaglandins are among the most important things in your life, and until now you had probably never heard of them. They were discovered in 1935 and are noted for their ability to cause some muscles to contract. Now, after much research scientists realize that the prostaglandins have a primary role in the onset and relief of inflammation.

TUG-OF-WAR

Inflammation is a tug-of-war phenomenon. On one side is one set of prostaglandins and other biochemicals that increases inflammation and on the other side a second group of prostaglandins and other biochemicals that suppresses or moderates inflammation. I think of the first group that initiate inflammation as "antagonistic" and the second group that moderate it as "beneficial."

Inflammation occurs when the antagonistic group is overpowering the beneficial group. My diet, however, helps to restore the balance. It strengthens the beneficial group. It helps to bring the situation closer to the neutral point.

Once you have restored the natural balance, if medication is necessary, it will be more effective.

THE BASIC PROBLEM

The prostaglandins are like hormones because they are made when required, balance is essential, and a very small amount of them goes a long way. Let me break that concept into some easy pieces.

Our body makes the prostaglandins instantaneously as required. This is in contrast to other biologically active materials, which are stored for a later date. For example, vitamins, enzymes, amino acids, fat, and carbohydrates are stored in most body tissues. Their presence in all body tissues is essential. The prostaglandins are different; only their building materials must be present so they can be made on demand.

The building blocks of the antagonistic prostaglandins are always readily available from your diet, but the building blocks of the beneficial prostaglandins are not.

ARACHIDONIC ACID AND THE ANTAGONISTIC PROSTAGLANDINS

Antagonistic prostaglandins are made from a fatty acid called arachidonic acid, which can be made from another fatty acid, linoleic acid. These fatty acids are plentiful in the American diet and one of them, linoleic acid, is actually essential in small quantities for health, because it serves as the building block for these and other materials.

Arachidonic acid is obtained from animal products. You get arachidonic acid whenever you eat animal fat. This includes meat, dairy products, and even egg yolks.

Linoleic acid is a plant fatty acid found in plant oils, such as corn oil, soybean oil, and other light vegetable oils. We also obtain some linoleic acid from meat and dairy products, because animals eat plants and store linoleic acid. But your major source is the oils used in cooking and in salads.

EPA AND THE BENEFICIAL PROSTAGLANDINS

Beneficial prostaglandins are made from a fatty acid found in marine plants and fish, named eicosapentaenoic acid—EPA, for short. EPA is not made by the fish; it is made by algae, plankton, and seaweed, which the fish eat. Because fish take on the temperature of their surroundings and EPA remains liquid at cold temperatures, it should be no surprise that cold-water fish accumulate EPA. Because big fish eat small fish, cold-water fish serve as a sort of a living factory that concentrates EPA beginning with seaweed.

EPA—ONE OF THREE OMEGA-3 FATTY ACIDS

EPA is the most important member of an exclusive group of three fatty acids, the "omega-3 fatty acids." This group includes alpha linolenic acid (ALA), eicosapentaenoic acid (EPA), and docosahexaenoic acid (DHA). Think of them as ALA, EPA, and DHA.

Omega-3 fatty acids are very exclusive members of a larger group of fatty acids, the polyunsaturated fatty acids. The omega-3 designation is important to chemists and health professionals because it identifies their special physical characteristics. We'll focus on the interrelation of them and on their importance to human health.

ALA

(Alpha Linolenic Acid)

ALA is made in the chloroplasts of green plants from another polyunsaturated fatty acid called linoleic acid. In mammals, linoleic acid is converted to arachidonic acid that is used to make the antagonistic prostaglandins. ALA is found in all green plants; this includes green vegetables, leaves, grass, algae, seaweed, and a myriad of others. Mammals, including humans, do not manufacture ALA.

ALA TO EPA

ALA is important because it serves as the building material for EPA. Fish, algae, plankton, and mammals, including man, convert ALA to EPA through normal metabolism. Fish and sea mammals (e.g., whales) eat the algae and plankton of the sea, accumulating EPA in their oily tissue. We either eat fish and get EPA or, through more recent modern engineering, remove it from the fish and put it in capsules that contain EPA.

Alternatively, when we consume animals such as deer, rabbits, and range animals (such as buffalo) we obtain some EPA because they accumulate it in their tissues, although not nearly as much as fish. Fish and sea mammals are rich sources of EPA because many of them live exclusively on plankton or eat other fish that do.

EPA TO DHA

DHA is an integral part of eye and brain tissue. Scientists are still studying the function of DHA in these tissues, but they all agree that DHA is important to the development and function of ocular tissue, brain tissue, and the tissue of other organs.

DHA is made by marine algae, plankton, fish, and mammals, including humans, from EPA. Fish accumulate DHA in their oily tissue, along with EPA.

WHY NOT SIMPLY EAT ALA?

Since our bodies can convert ALA to EPA, and similarly EPA to DHA, you might ask, Why not simply eat green plants for ALA and let our metabolism convert it to EPA and DHA?

While that seems logical and ALA conversion accounts for some of our EPA, it is a very inefficient way to get EPA, and especially inadequate for people with arthritis. We would not be able to eat enough green vegetables to satisfy our needs. But I must quickly point out that the more green vegetables we eat the better, because they provide many other important nutrients as well. However, we also need additional EPA. The conversion of ALA to EPA, albeit minor, helps us understand why vegetarian diets reduced the inflammation and pain of arthritis.

EPA IS KING

EPA is the most critical of the omega-3 fatty acids for arthritis. EPA is the only material that our bodies use to make the beneficial prostaglandins that help reduce inflammation. Most experts agree that one gram or more of EPA per day should be adequate.

Fish oils contain DHA and some ALA along with the EPA. This combination is important for another reason: the "push-pull" of metabolism. In the presence of DHA and ALA, all EPA can be converted to the beneficial prostaglandins rather than partially diverted for other uses. This is because sufficient DHA from the diet eliminates any need for additional DHA produced by the body. The EPA can be used to make the beneficial prostaglandins or stored for another time. Likewise, the presence of dietary ALA prevents any metabolic reversion that might convert EPA into ALA. Consequently, fish oil containing all omega-3 fatty acids is ideally suited for this diet.

GREENLANDERS' LESSON IN THE OMEGA-3 FATTY ACIDS

Some societies—for example, those of Greenlanders, Faeroe Islanders, seacoast villagers in Japan, and others—live on a rich fish diet and have a different balance of dietary fat than we do. They consume very little saturated fat and much more of the omega-3 fatty acids. For example, some of them get as much as 14 grams of the omega-3s daily. They also consume very little linoleic and arachidonic acids.

In contrast, the average American diet consists of much more saturated fat and arachidonic and linolcic acids, and we consume very little EPA, DHA, and ALA.

While the diet of the Greenlanders and others mentioned, helps them to have less heart disease, there are other benefits as well. Most of these benefits emerge as greatly reduced incidences of inflammatory diseases, which include arthritis. Not surprisingly, all these afflictions involve the balance between the beneficial and antagonistic prostaglandins. Indeed, the high fish diet gives an edge to the beneficial prostaglandins. In contrast, the average American diet gives a significant edge to the antagonistic prostaglandins. It's as simple as that.

PUTTING IT INTO PRACTICE

All this discussion on the omega-3 fatty acids and lessons from Greenlanders and others makes our mission for arthritis relief clear: decrease dietary linoleic and arachidonic acids, and increase EPA. The rewards are worth the effort and the diet provides many benefits.

CHAPTER
3 What Your Doctor Should Know

If your doctor is current on the latest findings in prostaglandin research, he or she will encourage you in your diet commitment. Many doctors know this diet can only help your arthritis and that it will benefit other conditions.

In contrast, your doctor might say that arthritis cannot be cured by diet, or that diet has nothing to do with arthritis. Indeed, nothing can cure arthritis. However, a chronic disease or condition does not exist that cannot benefit from proper diet. The science on which my plan is based is sound. It can do no harm and much good to everyone who follows it.

Most likely, this diet will be compatible with any course of medication your doctor is using; and of course, you should check with him. If you follow the diet consistently, it will support his efforts. This is the best type of doctor/patient teamwork I know. Both your objectives and your doctor's objectives come together in harmony.

THE NATURAL HARMONY STRATEGY

I think of the Arthritis Relief Diet as a "natural harmony strategy" because it uses all the body's natural resources to the best of their ability. If the diet isn't sufficient by itself, your physician can prescribe medication more effectively because your metabolism will be much more stable.

IMPORTANT EVIDENCE

I know this diet works for several reasons that should interest your doctor. First, we have had many people on an abbreviated version of my diet and their success is testimony to the approach. As one dieter put it so clearly, "I didn't know I could feel this good. I'm riding my bicycle again after twenty years."

Second, scientists have used it in several studies for various periods of time. Even the short-term success is remarkable. In these short-term studies lasting a month, it produced as much as 50% success and never less than 20%. Accumulated body fat serves as a source of arachidonic and linoleic acids, which makes short-term success less. The main source of EPA in these studies was supplementary EPA in capsules.

Other dietary approaches have used some of the same features. For example, total abstinence from food invariably produces short-term relief from arthritis. The reasons for this relief are twofold: The inducers of inflammation are removed and the precursers of the antagonistic prostaglandins are reduced.

Other societies, most notably the Chinese, have used a similar vegetarian diet for thousands of years. That approach, although somewhat successful because it reduced the antagonists, didn't restore the balance in favor of the beneficial prostaglandins even though it would surely have increased the alpha linolenic acid.

A third impressive body of evidence is unfolding in Greenland where inflammatory disease is much, much lower than in the United States. Thanks to computer capacity, epidemiologists can now explore the dietary differences in detail. Greenlanders have been an ongoing experiment of this diet for generations. They have been eminently successful.

A last body of evidence is indirect, but very important because it comes from research physicians. They have studied the effects of EPA on heart disease and related problems such as high blood pressure. In these studies they use a diet very similar to this one and use supplemental EPA. When asked if this diet results in any other effects, they note that the people on the study notice arthritis relief and the doctors themselves have often noticed a decrease in inflammation.

PART II

The Inflammation Fighters: Five Ways to Relieve Your Pain

CHAPTER
4 Inflammation Fighter #1: Excellent Protein Sources

Ten to 15% of the calories in your new diet will come from protein. If you're a typial American, you will automatically think of meat (i.e., beef—perhaps a nice thick steak—pork, or veal). Perhaps you even think of an omelet. The average person doesn't think of fish right away, even though it's the best source of protein available. A letter I recently received illustrates my point.

> *Dear Dr. Scala,*
>
> *I received your diet today and we were both delighted and disappointed. It's good news and bad news for us. The good news is that I'm sure it will work, but the bad news is that you recommend fish. The freezer is full of beef I've already got. We are a meat-eating family and my family agreed to make the commitment with me. So I will start cooking for myself, but they will have to start later.*

Most people think of protein as beef. In fact, each year the average American consumes 371 pounds of meat, 100 pounds of poultry, 239 pounds of eggs and milk, and only 36 pounds of fish. The preceding letter represents a typical response from a person who never eats fish, and only a little poultry. If

your major source of protein is meat, I want you to change
that pattern.

FISH IS BEST

By following my plan, you will change your eating habits so
that next year you will consume very little (if any) meat.
Instead, you will probably eat about 150 pounds or less of
poultry. Cutting back on milk and eggs with the exception of
skim milk and eggs in cooking will bring your egg and milk
consumption to less than 100 pounds. You will obtain excellent protein from vegetables, especially beans. Your fish consumption will increase to 150 pounds or more! And you will
feel great.

We need protein for growth, development, and body re-
newal. Just about all the foods we eat contain protein, but on
this plan fish, poultry, vegetables, and dairy products are the
major sources.

Did you know that 35% of the calories in mushrooms
comes from protein? Because there is no fat in mushrooms,
the remaining 65% of calories comes from excellent complex
carbohydrates, which include fiber.

In contrast to mushrooms, ground chuck gets 32% of its calories from protein and 66% of its calories from fat—lots of
arachidonic acid—and no carbohdyrate.

Compare that with a nice piece of salmon. Salmon delivers
67% of its calories from protein, 28% from fat with up to 1.5
grams of EPA. Eat just one meal of salmon each day, no
meat or animal products for the other two meals, and you will
feel better without doing anything else.

Fish provides the most protein for the least number of
calories and the best fat.

The following tables list some commonly consumed fish as a
function of serving size, calories, fat and, most important,
EPA content.

Total Polyunsaturated Fat Content of Commonly Available Fish*

Fish	Total Polyunsaturated (grams)
Tuna (canned in water)	3.0–5.0
Herring	2.6–5.0
Mackerel	2.6–5.0
Salmon (canned in water)	2.4–4.0
Rainbow trout	1.4–3.0
Flounder	0.4–1.0
Haddock	0.2–1.0

*Always expressed as grams per 3½-ounce serving.

EPA Content of Commonly Available Fish*

Fish	EPA Content per 3½-Ounce Serving (Grams)
Anchovy	0.7–1.5
Striped bass (fillet)	0.2–0.8
Cod (fillet)	0.3
Eel (fillet)	0.4–1.0
Flounder (fillet)	0.1–0.8
Herring	1.2–2.7
Halibut (fillet)	0.3
Mackerel	0.7–2.6
Sardines	0.9–1.0
Salmon (fillet)	1.0–2.6
Salmon (canned in water)	1.1–3.2
Salmon, coho	0.2–1.0
Snapper	0.1–0.3
Trout	0.2–1.0
Tuna (canned in water)	0.4–2.6
Whiting	0.9
Crab	0.6
Shrimp	0.5

*EPA content expressed as grams of EPA and alpha linolenic acid per 3½-ounce serving. The amount of EPA varies with the location of the catch, season, and the food the fish have been eating.

Fish can be classified several ways. This dietary commitment asks you to compare them on the basis of polyunsaturated fat content and EPA content. The following tables summarize both for you.

A SHORT REVIEW

This diet emphasizes low-fat protein. The protein in this diet is not simply adequate, it is excellent in both quantity and quality. Sources include fish, fowl, and vegetables. In short, any food that didn't swim, fly, or grow from the ground probably won't be good for you.

CHAPTER
5 Inflammation Fighter #2: Less Fat

Twenty to 25% of your calories should come from fat. If that number reaches 30%, you're still okay, but you should try harder.

On this diet you will minimize saturated animal fat and reduce your polyunsaturated oil intake. I want you to do this specifically to reduce arachidonic and linoleic acids. They are the primary substances from which the antagonistic prostaglandins are made, and we will strive to reduce them as much as possible.

You will also increase your EPA intake as much as possible. Remember, EPA is short for eicosapentaenoic acid, which we get from fish or as a food supplement. EPA is the substance from which the beneficial prostaglandins are made, and the objective of this plan is to get as much EPA as possible.

A FEW SIMPLE RULES

• Get at least 1 gram of EPA each day—in protein-rich fish and in capsules as food supplements; 2 grams would be better.

- Stop eating red meat from four-footed (hoofed) animals, and the dark meat of fowl.
- Stop using corn oil in cooking, frying, and baking. Instead use solid shortening such as butter if you must. When cooking with oil, use olive oil or Puritan oil. Olive oil is excellent for this diet. Puritan oil is rich in alpha linolenic acid even though it contains some linoleic acid. Other alternatives are soybean oil and peanut oil.
- Bake, broil, barbecue, boil, poach, microwave your food— even use a campfire if you can.
- Stop using egg yolks unless your serving provides a fraction of one egg. For example, a cake that uses one or two eggs and serves 10 to 16 pieces is okay. But just eat one piece!
- Stop using milk if it has fat in it. Skim milk and the products of skim milk are okay. Use yogurt or low-fat cottage cheese.

Learn to live with the preceding rules, and you will succeed. You will begin to feel relief as soon as you get into the plan.

Let's look at some foods you can eat to get the dietary fat you require.

Yes, you can eat all the fish you want. Some kinds of fish are better than others, but always remember, fish is best.

Poultry white meat is excellent as a protein source and it provides little fat. The only drawback is that it has no EPA.

A LESSON IN COOKING

We'll take a piece of chicken, a normal 3½-ounce breast, and prepare it two ways. I'll let you judge which is best.

Roast the chicken breast and it provides 166 calories; 126 calories or 76% of the total calories are from protein (32 grams or half your daily needs). Only 18% of calories come from fat. Even though chicken has no EPA, it's excellent for this plan. As a bonus, its low fat content makes it ideal for eliminating heart disease.

Now purchase the same piece of chicken from a typical fast-food emporium where it is breaded and cooked in fat under pressure. The same 3½ ounces now provides 323 calories of which 58% come from fat, 15% from the breading, and 27% from protein (22 grams).

There's more to this example. I used 3½ ounces in each case, so in the fast-food example, I reduced the protein by 10% to get the bread on it, then pumped it full of fat in the cooking. But more, the added fat is often (although not always) saturated fat from lard. It contains no EPA and much arachidonic acid, from which the antagonistic prostaglandins are made.

In both examples the chicken starts out with less than 200 milligrams of salt, and in the first example it stays that way or increases slightly if barbeque sauce is used. The fast-food example starts with less than 200 milligrams of salt, but it finishes with about 2,400 milligrams! Now you know what's in all those secret herbs, spices, and breading that are so tasty. Salt!

Fish and fowl are excellent sources of protein with little fat and they are balanced by nature. It's man who can either enhance them by broiling or barbequing or make them a metabolic nightmare by converting them to high-fat, high-salt foods.

EPA SUPPLEMENTS

Even if you decide to eat fish often, you may not get as much EPA as you want. The best sources of EPA are oily fishes such as mackerel and anchovies, but most people don't like them. Alternatives such as salmon, tuna, or trout are often unavailable or expensive. Other fish require two or more servings to get one gram of EPA. Like dietary supplements of vitamins and minerals, EPA capsules are actually food in capsule form. Thanks to modern engineering, the capsules are a convenient way to assure you of getting sufficient dietary EPA.

SUPPOSE YOU DON'T EAT FISH

If you think you can't eat fish, don't despair. Consult the many nonfish recipes in Chapter 12, and if your dietary EPA is still less than one gram per day, you can obtain insurance with EPA supplements.

But, I must urge you to try fish. It's a rare individual who cannot eat any fish. Learn which fishes agree with you and resolve to like them. Experiment with different recipes.

A SHORT REVIEW

This diet will provide adequate essential fats and emphasize EPA from fish and from supplements. A major dietary objective is to reduce total fat intake.

CHAPTER

6 Inflammation Fighter #3: Complex Carbohydrate

On my diet, 60 to 70% of your calories will come from carbohydrates.

As part of your commitment to controlling inflammation, you must increase your carbohydrate intake by emphasizing complex carbohydrates in your diet. Complex carbohydrates, in contrast to sugar, a simple carbohydrate, are those that nature provides in grains, cereals, tubers, vegetables, fruits, and leaves. We also consume complex carbohydrates such as pasta, whole-grain breads, cereals, and baked goods. It's what we do with what nature provides that counts.

Sugar, when not packaged by nature as fruit or other carbohydrate-rich food such as high-fiber cereal, high-fiber waffles, pancakes, and so on, gets into our bloodstream too quickly, and this may lead to mood swings and depression. Most experts claim it contributes to heart disease, diabetes, and other modern health problems.

Many American adults consume as much as 130 pounds of sugar per year, or a heaping 6-ounce glass full of sugar each day. Everyone says, "Not me!" In fact very few people use sugar directly. Most of us use less than 32 pounds of sugar directly per year; that's only 1.5 ounces each day, or little more than a teaspoon. Obviously, sugar is in all the processed food we eat. For example, the 8 fluid ounces of soft drinks we average each day contain almost 7 teaspoons. Bread, desserts, and fast foods contain sugar. It is everywhere, even in salami, which I implore you not to eat.

BLOOD SUGAR AND YOUR MOODS

Sugar entering our blood too quickly causes a rapid increase in blood sugar. Our body responds to the rapid increase by producing insulin, a hormone that facilitates utilization of the sugar. When the sugar is excessive, the insulin response is excessive, and within a short time the blood sugar drops below normal because of the excess insulin. This produces a condition known as "hypoglycemia," which means low blood sugar.

Blood sugar influences our moods. After all, it's the only energy source our brain has available, and when it's too low it's a sort of primitive signal that all is not well. This leads to a number of mood changes, which range from irritable and anxious to depressed. Because 18% of people with arthritis suffer from depression, it's important to monitor your blood sugar level. The rule is simple: Don't use sugar or foods that contain a lot of sugar.

A SHORT REVIEW

On this diet, carbohydrates will account for 60% or more of your caloric intake.

Emphasis is placed on the complex, natural carbohydrates found in fruit, vegetables, grains, and pastas.

The plan helps to maintain constant blood sugar levels.

CHAPTER

7 Inflammation Fighter #4: Dietary Fiber

Your new diet will include 25 to 35 grams, or at least 1 ounce of dietary fiber each day with the carbohydrate-rich foods and as fiber supplements.

Our bodies produce many materials that get eliminated in a number of ways. Some get excreted in the urine and others in the intestinal tract by way of the gallbladder or through the intestine itself. The important thing is that the system have available adequate dietary fiber to bind up these materials and flush them from the body.

I'm always asked, "How much fiber do I require?" and my answer is, "So you have a bowel movement every 24 hours."

You get this fiber by eating high-fiber cereal, grains, vegetables, fruit, high-fiber bread, and by thoughtful supplementation. You cannot get too much dietary fiber. I've done lots of studies on dietary fiber, I've seen lots of studies on dietary fiber, and in twenty years I've never encountered a situation in which people have gotten too much dietary fiber.

But if you must be precise, the experts teach that we should get from 25 to 35 grams each day; that's a little over 1 ounce of dietary fiber. One ounce of dietary fiber requires that you eat lots of fruit, cereal, grains, and vegetables daily.

In nutrition, teamwork is important and the team member

of fiber is water. Water is another nutrient that's hard to take to excess. Fiber can bind you up if you don't get enough water to go with it. After all, fiber is the plant material that binds water. And, in the presence of water, fiber makes your stool soft but consistent. In the absence of water it can make them dry and hard.

You can understand the relationship between water and fiber more clearly by this analogy. Milk contains less water than green peas. The reason you don't eat milk with a fork and drink your peas is the fiber in peas; it gives peas their shape and holds the water. You want it to do exactly that in your digestive system: Give stools consistency without firmness.

Hard fiber, the type found in wheat bran, is the "water carrier" that helps to produce regularity. It gives good stool consistency and achieves the objective of regularity. This fiber is found in all plant food, but mostly in the high-fiber cereals, the grains, most vegetables, beans, and tubers such as potatoes. You can't eat too much of these foods and the results will be obvious as you increase them in your diet.

THE SELECTIVE CARRIER

I said fiber is like a brush with selective bristles which, in addition to moving things along, can selectively bind unwanted materials and remove them from the system. Put another way, there are about five or six types of fiber, all of which have properties we require. And a varied diet provides them all. Sometimes selective supplementation helps.

In contrast to the hard fiber, the soluble forms of fiber seem to be the best at selective absorption. For example, pectin helps to reduce cholesterol by binding the bile acids produced by our liver from cholesterol and removing them in our stools. Oat bran does it even better—and guar gum even better yet. It also binds the cholesterol and fat that we get in our diet and helps to carry them through the system.

Not surprising there's evidence that selective dietary fiber can help to remove by-products of metabolism, which helps arthritics. It appears that some materials produced by the body and secreted into the intestine by the gallbladder act as antagonists, and cause arthritis inflammation. Also, from the results of intestinal bypass surgery, it is obvious that the microflora of the intestine can do the same thing.

A famous study used fiber from the desert plant yucca and observed the same result. But before you rush out and purchase either yucca fiber or alfalfa tablets, remember, we are getting involved in a complete diet plan and our objective is a total commitment.

FIBER FROM FOOD

An easy way to get a good start on the fiber you need is to begin each day with high-fiber cereal. Many excellent cereals are available; All-Bran, Bran Buds, Bran Flakes, Corn Bran, Oat Bran, oatmeal, and barley, to name a few. Add unprocessed bran to pancakes or waffles. Eat fruit on cereal, in pancakes, or plain; eat fruit and more fruit along with vegetables, grains, and tubers at each meal. As your fiber intake improves, you'll become more regular.

High-fiber snacks are excellent all day, but drink lots of water. Water increases the value of fiber. The following list contains some readily available cereals that provide sufficient dietary fiber.

COLD CEREALS

Over 12 grams dietary fiber per serving:

- Kellogg's All-Bran Extra Fiber
- General Mills Fiber One

9 grams of dietary fiber:

- Kellogg's All-Bran
- Nabisco 100% Bran

3 to 5 grams of fiber:

- Quaker Corn Bran
- Ralston Bran Chex
- Kellogg's Raisin Bran
- Generic or store brand raisin bran
- Kellogg's Cracklin' Oat Bran
- Kellogg's Bran Flakes
- General Mills Raisin Nut Bran
- Post Fruit 'N Fiber
- Post Bran Flakes
- Post Natural Raisin Bran

HOT CEREALS

- Quaker Oats
- Malt-O-Meal Co. Hot Wheat Cereal
- Ralston Cream of Wheat
- Wheatena
- Bran. Unprocessed Bran
- Miller unprocessed Bran
- Quaker unprocessed Bran

FIBER SUPPLEMENTS

Most fiber supplements that you mix with water are made from psyllium seed. It provides musilage, which helps to bulk the stools and maintain regularity. Other fiber snacks, such as fiber wafers and high-fiber crackers and cookies, are also fiber supplements that are simply eaten as food.

WATER

Fiber cannot perform its cleansing action without water. But, our requirement for water extends far beyond its teamwork with fiber. Indeed, next to air itself, it is the most important of all nutrients. In arthritis it is especially important for the elimination of waste materials that, in the opinion of some experts, can cause flare-ups.

Strive for eight glasses of water daily. Although it is best if consumed as pure water, it is okay in the form of other beverages as well.

A SHORT REVIEW

Fiber can help arthritis and contribute to general health. This diet includes lots of fiber.

Fiber is obtained from cereals, grains, fruits, and vegetables. It is also available in supplement form.

There are many types of fiber and all are important for this diet to be effective. Therefore I emphasize variety.

Water is necessary as a nutrient and as a teamworker with fiber. Drink lots of water.

8 Inflammation Fighter #5: Nutrient Balance

In addition to protein, fat, carbohydrates, and fiber, your body requires nineteen vitamins and minerals daily to function normally. These requirements are expressed in terms of the recommended daily allowance, or RDA for short. Most of them are required in very small quantities; for example, some, like folic acid, in microgram quantities; most, like iron, in milligram quantities; and a few, like sodium and calcium, in excess of 1,000 milligrams each day.

On this diet plan you'll get adequate amounts of most nutrients, excepting perhaps calcium, magnesium, and iron, because of our avoidance of milk and meat. I don't believe in leaving anything to chance, and therefore recommend you insure our diet with supplementation to avoid any possible marginal deficiencies.

VITAMIN-MINERAL SUPPLEMENTATION

"Nutrition insurance" is an overworked slogan. But, in my arthritis plan, the phrase is appropriate. I would like to supplement your diet with from one-half (50%) to one time (100%) of the RDA for all nineteen vitamins and minerals. Why only one-half to one time the RDA for vitamins and minerals? This diet plan will supply the RDA for most of the required nutrients, but our major dietary objective is to reduce inflammation and, as a result, a little variety is lost and some nutrients, such as iron, magnesium, calcium, and a few others will fall short. Supplementation is an easy way of insuring that the nutrients are present in adequate supply and any excess will be insurance. A few examples might help.

Adult women require 800 to 1,000 milligrams of calcium each day up to about age 50, and then most nutritionists believe that calcium intake should be elevated to 1,200 or 1,500 milligrams. Because milk is the most common source of calcium, that translates into 3½ to 5½ glasses of milk or calcium-rich food like yogurt each day. A serving of broccoli or spinach provides the calcium of a half glass of milk, together with other nutrients. So you should ask yourself if you consume sufficient dairy products each day. If not, common sense says to use a calcium supplement.

Iron is another good example. A typical diet contains about 6 milligrams of iron for each 1,000 calories. Women require 18 milligrams of iron each day. That translates to 3,000 calories. But the rub is that most women don't consume more than 2,000 calories each day, hence the shortfall. After menopause, a woman's iron requirement drops to that of men—10 milligrams a day. To add insult to injury, research indicates that some arthritics do not absorb iron as effectively as they should; therefore making sure of enough is simply common sense.

Vitamin C is one of the most abused vitamins we know. The government recommends 65 milligrams each day and other often self-appointed nutritionists recommend up to several grams. Medications used in the treatment of arthritis sometimes destroy vitamin C. Therefore getting enough is an important consideration.

Although the debate will continue for many years, fresh fruits and vegetables, our best sources of vitamin C, are often lacking, especially in senior citizens. So practicality says we should get more vitamin C. And I believe the RDA should be about 200 to 300 milligrams.

Rather than go through each nutrient, for the reasons I have discussed, the diet of the arthritic is on the average not as good as the diet of the general public who don't have arthritis. And because the general public usually falls a little short on many nutrients, logic teaches that people with arthritis fall short as well.

A BASIC SUPPLEMENT

I propose that you use a supplement that provides the vitamins and minerals listed in the following tables.

Nutrient Vitamin	Amount per Tablet*	Percent U.S. RDA
Vitamin A	2,500 I.U.**	50
Vitamin D	200 I.U.	50
Vitamin E	15 I.U.	50
Vitamin C	30 mg.	50
Folic acid	0.2 mg.	50
Thiamin (B1)	0.75 mg.	50
Riboflavin (B2)	0.86 mg.	50
Niacin	10. mg.	50
Vitamin B6	1. mg.	50
Vitamin B12	3. micrograms	50
Biotin	0.15 mg.	50
Pantothenic acid	5. mg	50

*Two tablets provide 100% U.S. RDA.
**International Units

Nutrient Minerals	Amount per Tablet	Percent U.S. RDA
Calcium**	0.5 grams	50
Phosphorus**	0.4 grams	40
Iodine	75. micrograms	50
Iron	9. mg.	50
Magnesium	200. mg.	50
Copper	1. mg.	50
Zinc	1. mg.	50
Selenium	50. micrograms	50

*See text for calcium and phosphorus. Also, get calcium level to 0.5
**Two tablets provide 100% U.S. RDA.
†International Units.

Few products satisfy the preceding criteria. Usually the product you select will not have sufficient calcium, phosphorus, or magnesium. If it doesn't, do not worry because you should take extra calcium anyway. Your diet already contains excess phosphorus and provides about 50% of the magnesium you need. If the product you select comes to within 10 to 20% of each nutrient listed above, it is fine. Don't select a supplement that varies by more than that amount. Most products that meet my criteria are labeled to deliver 100% of the U.S. RDA in a two-tablet serving. Some require a four-tablet serving.

Shaklee Vita-Lea meets the requirement most completely. If used with this diet, you only require additional calcium or calcium and magnesium. Other products exceed some of the vitamins, but fall short in minerals, especially calcium and magnesium.

Read the nutritional label carefully and be sure the product you select is balanced.

Calcium will be required in addition to the basic supplement program. Strive to get 1,000 milligrams of calcium daily if you're below age 50 and 1,200 milligrams if you're above age 50. That's about four to six glasses of milk and lots of dark green vegetables. But because I ask you to avoid dairy products such as milk and cheese on this diet, it is appropriate to take three calcium supplements of about 250 milligrams each day.

B COMPLEX

Some people feel better if they use the B complex vitamins as a supplement over and above the basic supplement I recommend. The B vitamins are those listed on the basic supplement as folic acid, thiamine (B1), riboflavin (B2), niacin, vitamin B6 (sometimes listed as pyridoxal phosphate), vitamin B12, and biotin. If you wish to take more B vitamins, always take them together as a supplement containing all the B vitamins balanced in the same RDA levels and never more than 500% (or five times) of the RDA in a single tablet.

SPECIAL SUPPLEMENTS OF SINGLE NUTRIENTS

There is a continuing debate surrounding vitamins E, C, and a newly recognized, but old nutrient, beta-carotene, zinc, and a few others.

Vitamin C The debate ranges from those who advocate up to 10 grams per day, to those who advise caution and no more than the U.S. RDA of 65 milligrams. This debate has precipitated much discussion among experts, and will probably continue into the next century. The lack of resolution has to do with the criteria on which RDAs are established. Not long ago, the deficiency disease of vitamin C was scurvy, but now we are considering such heavy issues as its effect in preventing cancer, and scurvy pales in comparison.

In the past, it was suggested that vitamin C has some specific relationship to arthritis. We know today that it does not, but we understand how this misconception developed. In the development of scurvy, one of the early symptoms is swelling of the joints, especially the knees, which was actually called "arthritis." This was the result of a breakdown of tissue from the deficiency, and not the arthritis we know.

Anyone who uses aspirin regularly requires more vitamin C. Aspirin destroys vitamin C in the body and increases the dietary need when people use it or similar more modern medications.

This diet plan provides from 100 to 300 milligrams of vitamin C, depending on your use of fruits, vegetables, and grains. There is certainly no harm and, in my opinion, probably much good in using an additional vitamin C supplement up to 500 milligrams. I believe the human vitamin C requirement is significantly higher than the present RDA of 65 milligrams.

Vitamin E does not have any effect on arthritis beyond its importance in general good health. From time to time reports have surfaced to the contrary, but none with any scientific support.

The vitamin E requirement is related to polyunsaturated fat intake. If you follow this diet plan and use the basic supplement, you should exceed the vitamin E RDA by as much as 50%.

Other health problems do produce a vitamin E requirement of 600 I.U. or more daily. These are not related to arthritis and involve therapeutic uses of the vitamin.

Selenium is a trace mineral that is generally deficient in people with arthritis.

This dietary plan assures you of adequate selenium, which is obtained in fruits, vegetables, and grains. By eating a variety of fresh foods you obtain ample selenium—and, for insurance, use the supplement described in this chapter.

Old folk-wisdom teaches that we should eat an apple a day. Although the originator of that advice didn't specifically have selenium in mind, he or she could have, because apples are a good source of selenium.

Zinc During the question session of a lecture I gave in Indianapolis, I was asked if there were any dangers from zinc intakes of ten times the RDA. I cited studies which indicate that ten times the RDA of zinc can cause a copper deficiency and a shift in cholesterol, which is not good. A week later I received a letter from a physician, asking why his patient had wanted to stop the high zinc intake he had prescribed to treat her rheumatoid arthritis. I advised him that his patient had disregarded my advice: the use of supplements to correct dietary shortfall is not applicable to patients who are taking high therapeutic levels of dietary and mineral supplements under a doctor's care.

Dietary studies have indicated that arthritis sufferers often have inadequate zinc in their diets. But this is because their diets lack variety, especially fish. There is no indication that people with arthritis should self-medicate with zinc. Taking zinc at ten times the RDA is the domain of the physician. This plan and the recommended supplement will provide adequate zinc.

Beta-carotene is the vegetable precurser of vitamin A; consequently, our body converts beta-carotene to vitamin A as it is required for bodily function. Studies of dietary adequacy usually indicate that most people, especially those over 50, get less Vitamin A or beta-carotene than they require. This diet should be adequate in beta-carotene, especially if you use the general supplement plan. If you do not feel secure in your consumption of vegetables, however, supplemental beta-carotene can provide nutritional insurance.

EPA This dietary plan balances the prostaglandins, depending heavily on dietary EPA. Eskimos obtain up to 14 grams of EPA daily! Some evidence suggests that they could be getting an excess. There is no danger of consuming such massive amounts on this diet, and there is much evidence indicating that 3 to 4 grams daily is safe and adequate.

Although evidence suggests that we should strive for 3 to 4

grams of EPA daily, I would like to see everyone get at least 1 gram. You can achieve 1 or more grams by choosing enough of the proper fish. Your insurance is the use of supplemental EPA.

EPA SUPPLEMENTS

EPA supplements are relatively new, so care must be taken in how you use them. Divide 1,000 by the number of milligrams of EPA in each capsule to get the number of capsules necessary to obtain 1 gram.

For example, suppose your EPA capsules contain 180 milligrams of EPA and weigh 650 milligrams each. Therefore 1,000 divided by 180 yields 6, which is the number of capsules necessary to get 1 gram (1,000 milligrams) of EPA.

Some other capsules contain more EPA, but beware of the size of the capsule. A 650-milligram capsule is comfortable to swallow, whereas a 1,000-milligram capsule is too large for many people. And one or two extra small capsules is easier to use than one large one.

Most EPA is sold as a concentrate from fish oil, which contains DHA as well. DHA (short for docosahexaenoic acid) is also an important nutrient, but has no known effect on either arthritis or other inflammatory problems. DHA does have an important role in the metabolism of EPA. This is discussed in Chapter Two.

Don't be confused by the size of the capsule or the percentage concentration. Simply look for the EPA content in milligrams per capsule and take enough to get 1 gram or more each day.

ALFALFA

When one person tells his doctor, "I feel better when I use alfalfa," it's an isolated experience. When many people relate the same experience, we say it's "anecdotal" evidence. That means it's not obtained from a well-designed study, but from cumulative human experience. Such evidence can often be valuable. On the one hand, it can lead to understanding the role of particular dietary components, and it can also focus attention on serious problems, such as dangerous side-effects.

People have used alfalfa for thousands of years, beginning with the Egyptians and Arabs. Today, people take alfalfa supplements made from dried leaves of mature plants. Folklore teaches that alfalfa works somewhat like aspirin. But in fact, alfalfa does not inhibit the production of antagonistic prostaglandins the way aspirin does.

Alfalfa, like many other vegetable foods, contains fiber. My theory is that fiber helps remove materials that induce inflammation from the intestinal tract. This concept is not new: Hippocrates himself suggested that constipation aggravated arthritis. More recently, some physicians have aggressively advocated high-fiber diets for people with arthritis as well. If this theory is correct, the beneficial effect attributed to alfalfa is due to the fact that it contains fiber, rather than to any specific pharmacologically active substance.

At present, evidence of benefits of alfalfa use is largely anecdotal. But one study, conducted on fiber extracted from another plant with a similar history of folk use, supports my theory. I anxiously await future developments.

GAMMA LINOLENIC ACID (GLA)

One other group of prostaglandins is derived from a fatty acid, gamma linolenic acid (GLA for short). Because our body can make GLA from dietary linoleic acid, dietary analysis suggests that there is no need for supplemental GLA, which can be obtained from seeds such as cottonseed and linseed.

It has been proposed, but never proven, however, that some people lack the metabolic ability to convert linoleic acid to GLA in sufficient quantity; hence its proposed use as a supplement for some people.

There is some scientific evidence indicating the GLA can be of help as a therapeutic agent in problems not related to arthritis. And some animal studies have suggested that it can help to slow the inflammatory response if induced by certain mildly toxic agents.

Therefore GLA falls into the realm of materials that are purported to have an effect with little scientific or anecdotal support. If your body makes GLA adequately, this plan will supply sufficient linoleic acid for the purpose.

ADDITIONAL SUPPLEMENTS?

Food supplementation grew slowly in the United States, beginning in the late 1920s and 1930s. They range from the modest multivitamin-multimineral supplement, which I recommend as a foundation, to all types of single supplements and combinations of various nutrients.

People use other supplements because they make them feel better. I can only propose that you give this diet and its recommended foundation of supplementation a good chance. Although I do not have a scientific basis to believe that additional supplementation will make the diet work better, I similarly cannot say that additional supplementation will make it not work. I do, however, advise caution.

A SHORT REVIEW

This diet is nutritionally sound with the exception of moderate shortfalls in iron, calcium, magnesium, and a few vitamins. People with arthritis may require more of these nutrients.

Supplementation is emphasized as the means of insuring your general diet and meeting those additional needs.

PART III

The Diet: Your Lifetime Nutrition Plan

CHAPTER
9 You're in Control

Food selection is your personal responsibility. An enormous variety of food is available to you within this plan. You only have to select food within the categories I've established, and the objective will take care of itself. What is the objective? To reduce the inflammation to a minimum!

The foods you should eat I call the *Do's*. Foods you should never eat again I call the *Don'ts*. And, similarly, foods you can eat *Occasionally*. I have also listed some *Caution* foods for your personal experimentation.

I want you to realize that you are in complete control of your own destiny. It's up to you to keep track of what, when, why, and how you feel, and to make positive adjustments. In the next few chapters I will suggest foods, menus, and recipes, but the choice of what specifically to eat at any given time is yours.

START TODAY

While you follow this diet plan you will get in much closer touch with your body and its relationship to food than ever before. I'm sure you want to begin as quickly as possible. Starting a food diary is the best way to jump right in.

A practical way is to purchase a small spiral notebook, preferably about 5 × 7, to fit into a pocket, purse, or briefcase: Record *what* you eat and drink, *how much, when,* and *why.* Then, at the beginning of each day, note briefly how you feel; for example, inflammation, morning stiffness in hands, ability to grip something, pain, and so on, and try to compare it with how you felt the previous morning. Do the same in the evening, but also evaluate your food in one or two sentences— was it good for you, was it balanced, did you eat enough or too much?

Just as each journey—no matter how long—starts with the first step, each life accounts for an enormous amount of food, each taken one bite at a time. You are now going to make each bite work for you.

HOW THE DIARY WORKS

You'll probably discover that inflammation comes with some foods and that it can be reduced by other foods. Then, you can eliminate those foods that are antagonistic and increase those that are beneficial. You will start to feel results as food supplements make it easy to get the nutrients that have the greatest benefit.

The benefit of keeping a food diary was vividly illustrated by an experiment I conducted with a group of students that wanted to lose weight. The professor introduced me and told them I was doing some research on food habits and would like each of them to keep a food diary. Each was given a pocket diary in which they listed everything they ate or drank, how much, when, and why. Then, each night before retiring, they were required to spend 10 minutes reviewing what foods they had eaten and write a short 25-word summary of their review.

Every member of that group lost weight; they are slender to this day and are among the most food-conscious people I know. They also enjoy all the food they eat. They never went on a diet. Each of them told me that the act of having to think through what they ate forced them to take control of themselves. They each recognized on their own what they could do to control their eating habits while still enjoying food. They developed new habits without ever consciously dropping old habits.

CALL TO ACTION

I've given you an assignment: Start a food diary. Do it now!

There is no special way to keep a food diary. Just write what, when, why, and how you feel about your food. Do it every day—no matter what you eat.

Get in touch with how you feel.

Here is a sample entry from the diary I keep myself:

Date: May 13

MORNING

What: All-Bran, ½ banana, skim milk, two cups of tea with skim milk and sweetener

When: About 8:00 A.M.—I feel great

Why: Feeling hungry after writing all morning—starting at 5:30 A.M. Broke at 7:00 A.M. to exercise.

What: Cup of tea, supplements (Vita-Lea, vitamin C, one B complex, six EPA, one beta-carotene)

When: About 10:00 A.M.

Why: As a snack after a phone call from National Nutritional Ed. Soc.

AFTERNOON

What: Tuna sandwich, lemon juice, Egg Beater mayonnaise, apple, a cup of tea with sweetener and milk

When: About 12:30 P.M.

Why: Hungry. Just finished writing a chapter. Good time to break before going to my boat to varnish the cap rails and to order a new #24 winch for the mast.

What: Tea with sweetener and skim milk and an apple

When: 3:45 P.M. with Bill Patience—just talking

Why: To take a break and pass the time pleasantly before my search for new winch

EVENING

What: Baked red snapper, normal serving, salad, string beans, Italian bread, fruit pudding, tea as usual, and an apple

When: About 7:30 P.M.

Why: Dinner with Nancy, Kim, and Greg; we planned our Memorial Day cruise from San Francisco to Half Moon Bay.

Critique: This was a good day. I feel fine. I'm going to try not to use sweeteners in my tea. No aches, no pain.

You can do better with your own diary. I know you can! So go ahead. I have seen people adopt many types of diaries; some have used commercial daytime planners, others have used elaborate computer recorders. Try whatever works for you. But remember that three things are absolutely essential—honesty, keeping track of everything you eat, and paying attention to the results. Your end-of-the-day critique is the most important step of all. If done correctly, it will give you a better understanding of yourself and your relationship to food.

CHAPTER
10 Fourteen Essential Do's, Don'ts, and Cautions

1. DON'T MISS OUT ON THE REWARDS

These *Do's* and *Don'ts* are your guide to reducing inflammation, so the first *Don't* is *Don't* deviate from the guidelines. The rewards will be great. You will get a new lease on life within a few weeks. So go at it with enthusiasm and vigor.

2. DO READ LABELS AS YOU SHOP

There are from 8,000 to 14,000 different items in your supermarket, depending upon its size. New selections are added each week and others disappear. So how can I tell you what to buy? I can show you how to read labels, that's how!

Food labels should provide two very important panels of information—the ingredient list and the nutritional information panel; the format of each is established by the Food and Drug Administration. Therefore once you catch on, they are all approximately the same.

The ingredient list must contain all the ingredients in descending order of content by weight. Once you get to the third or fourth ingredient, most of the others are not in sufficient quantity to count; thus we'll focus on the first three or four. Nutritional label panels carry information about calories, protein, fat, carbohydrate, and vitamin-mineral content as a function of the U.S. RDA. Most products now also contain information on sodium and dietary fiber.

I want to take you through one food product to illustrate these points:

Raisin Bran Cereal

Ingredients: Whole wheat, wheat bran, raisins, sugar
This ingredient list tells us that the product is fine for our purposes; it is, in fact, a fairly natural cereal. The nutritional panel will tell us more. It tells us that a serving is 1 ounce, which is about ½ cup. It lays out the following:

	1 Ounce of Cereal	With ½ Cup of Whole Milk
Calories	90	160 (130 skim)
Protein	2	6
Carbohydrate	22	28
Fat	0	4 (1 skim)
Sodium	160	220

Then the panel contains all this, together with the vitamins and minerals. And at the bottom of the panel it shows that the product delivers 4 grams of dietary fiber for each serving of ½ cup.

This short lesson can provide more information if you are willing to multiply the fat in grams by 9 to get total calories from fat and divide by the total calories to get the percentage from fat.

Raisin bran with whole milk gives 36 calories from fat; that's 23% of calories. Therefore it would be okay to use it on our diet plan, but it would be better with low-fat milk and even better with skim milk to avoid the fat completely. In fact, it would be ideal to use skim milk with double the cereal to get 8 grams of fiber.

Spaghetti often contains no formal ingredient list because it is made only from durum wheat, and there is no artificial coloring or salt added.

The nutritional label shows that in a serving of 2 ounces dry weight, you get 210 calories, 7 grams protein, 41 grams (1½ ounces) of carbohydrate, and only 1 gram of fat (less than 4% of calories).

If the sauce is selected with care, you will have a meal with adequate protein, high in complex carbohydrate, and almost devoid of fat. An excellent selection!

Egg Beaters' ingredient list looks complex but is actually very simple; 99% of the product is egg white and the remaining 1% creates the artificial yolk from corn oil and vegetable gums, which are a form of fiber and color.

The nutritional label tells you that the product compares very favorably with eggs for nutritional delivery without the fat content of the egg yolk—especially the cholesterol.

From this brief review you can see that by reading labels you can select packaged food wisely. In this way, once you become experienced, you can move through a supermarket very quickly.

CHEMICAL-SOUNDING NAMES

At the end of most ingredient lists are the materials used in minute amounts. These are things such as erythroborate, EDTA, hydroxybutylated toluene, propionic acid, monosodium glutamate, and many others, including some coloring agents. I cannot say they are unsafe, because if they had been proven unsafe, they would be outlawed; however, I still try to avoid them.

I avoid them because food safety is not a firm concept. In my career I have known of additives that were safe until a new, more sensitive test was devised, and now they are no longer allowed. I advise you to use caution and eat natural foods.

3. USE CAUTION WITH NIGHTSHADE PLANTS

The nightshade plants are controversial in arthritis. It is speculated that there is something in them that induces the immune system to attack. This attack translates into inflammation and pain. But it doesn't happen to everyone who has arthritis, in fact not many people at all. So there's probably some type of food sensitivity involved, which simply affects more people than average. Therefore I urge you to explore these foods for yourself. Hopefully you can use them, because they are excellent nourishment and are worth more than one serious try.

Testing is easy; simply make a note in your food diary whenever you use one of them and then avoid them for three or four days. If you get a reaction, an inflamed or sore joint, usually within 8 hours, you will know to avoid that food. Caution must also guide you to be sure that something else didn't cause one reaction, such as a weather change or some other stress. Try it one more time.

The nightshade foods are as follows:

Tomatoes: Yes, the old standby of so much cooking and so many cuisines.
Potatoes: Most varieties of white potatoes fall into the nightshade family. Therefore each variety should be tested. And be sure to use them with and without skin. Sweet potatoes are not nightshade plants and are an excellent source of both carbohydrate and fiber.
Eggplant: There are many varieties of eggplant. The most common is the purple-skinned eggplant. Test them all.

Peppers: The pepper comes in many varieties, ranging from the green mild variety to the hot reds that burn your mouth. I think you should test peppers before rejecting any of them, unless you simply don't like the hot, spicy variety.

The majority of the remainder of the plants in this family are either ornamental or are used as drugs and herbs and are of no concern to us.

I believe that most people who suffer from arthritis are not sensitive to these plants. This is from experience, not science. Therefore give them a serious try because they expand the breadth of your eating horizons and are excellent, nourishing foods.

4. DO EAT LOTS OF FISH

When you become a "fisharian," your life will change for the better.

Chapter 4 lists fish in descending order of EPA content, and you can get the basic idea from the following list. Strive for 3 to 4 grams of EPA each day, with 1 gram as a minimum. Remember the Eskimos consume about 14 grams of EPA each day.

For example, one 3.5-ounce serving of white-meat albacore tuna contains 1.7 grams of EPA, your daily basic requirement with room to spare in a modest serving. Canned bluefin tuna contains 0.9 grams in a 3.5-ounce serving, however, but 5 ounces provides over 1.3 grams—that's enough. Take a couple of EPA capsules as insurance and you're home free.

The general rule with fish is that some is always better than none. Fish with blue skin is best and the colder the water it lives in, the better.

When selecting a fish steak (e.g., from tuna, swordfish, or salmon), always select the steak closest to the head; it's richer in EPA.

EPA* Content of Fish at a Glance

Finfish	Total EPA grams/3½-oz. serving
High Fat Fish Mackerel Sable fish	0.9 to 2.6 grams
Medium Fat Fish Salmon Trout Whitefish	grams/3 ½-oz. serving 0.3 to 2.0 grams
Low-fat Fish Bass Cod Flounder Sole	grams/3 ½-oz. serving 0.1 to 1.0 grams

*Total EPA and alpha linolenic acid

Frozen Fish Is Fine

Modern fishing fleets have shipboard facilities to freeze fish whole or immediately after filleting or cutting into steaks. Although fish frozen this way never tastes quite as good as fresh, it comes very close. Moreover, these fresh frozen fish are better than fresh fish, which have been "fresh" for a week or two. Use frozen fish, fish fillets, or fish steaks as often as you can. I do not want you to use prepackaged, breaded frozen fish.

Canned Fish

Select fish packed in brine if possible; if not, drain off the oil; usually soy oil is used and is better than corn oil. But, canned tuna and salmon are very good sources of EPA and the cost is much less than fresh. Besides, they make excellent sandwiches. Don't prepare them with mayonnaise only—use

Egg Beater mayonnaise or a little olive oil, some lemon juice, and learn to enjoy the taste of the fish. In Chapter 12, "Basic Recipes," there is a recipe for preparing canned fish for a sandwich or salad as well as Egg Beater mayonnaise.

NONFIN FISH: MOLLUSKS, CRUSTACEANS, AND CEPHALOPODS

Mollusks (oysters, clams, etc.), crustaceans (shrimp, crabs, etc.), and cephalopods (squid, octopus, etc.) contain EPA but less than fin fish; in short, they are not good sources of EPA. You can assume they contain less than ½ gram per 3½-ounce serving. Use supplementary EPA when nonfin fish are the only seafood on your menu.

A Word About Cholesterol

Most shellfish contain cholesterol. In fact, most flesh, whether from fish, fowl, or four-legged animals contains cholesterol. But shellfish, especially mollusks, have been erroneously given the reputation of being high in cholesterol. Actually they don't contain as much cholesterol as people think; in fact, they are about the same as fish and fish is definitely a low-cholesterol food. The misunderstanding occurred because mollusks contain materials that are similar to cholesterol—sterols—which chemists have often labeled as cholesterol. With more sophisticated scientific techniques, however, we know now it is not. On the contrary, these sterols help reduce cholesterol.

Shrimp, crab, lobster, more specifically crustaceans, in contrast to mollusks, do contain cholesterol. They don't contain as much as eggs, but they do contain about 150 to 200 milligrams per 3½-ounce serving. Who eats only 3½ ounces of lobster? I urge you to keep your dietary cholesterol down, but

if shrimp, lobster, and crab are your major sources of cholesterol, economics will likely prevail and you will not be able to
afford them often enough to do any harm. In addition, there
is some evidence that their low fat level probably outweighs
the cholesterol content.

The extra fiber you will be getting from cereals, fruits, and
vegetables will help to reduce your blood cholesterol. So, if
you can afford them, go ahead and eat shrimp, crab, and
lobster, but think of the rest of us as you enjoy your meal.

Cooking the "Do" Fish

Broil, bake, and poach are the methods of choice for preparing fish on this plan. But, if you wish to fry, do so with
olive oil or Puritan oil. Grudgingly, I will allow soybean oil,
cottonseed oil, almond, and peanut oil as alternatives.

Breading can be done with whole-grain dried bread crumbs
or oatmeal to increase fiber intake. If breading requires milk,
use skim milk; if breading requires eggs, use egg whites or
Egg Beaters—not egg yolks. Chapter 12 contains basic fish-
breading recipes.

A Word About Garlic and Onions

Garlic and onions impart flavor to anything, especially fish,
and can make a plain meal an eating adventure. In addition,
garlic and onions contain chemical compounds that help this
plan produce better results (these are discussed under "Garlic, Onions, etc." later in this chapter). Use garlic and onions;
they're great for flavor and health!

Watch Out!

Don't eat fish from the various fast-food emporiums. This
plan is all about fish as God made them. But what God has
made, man can put asunder. And man puts it asunder by

deep-fat frying, usually in animal fat. I'm thinking of the square fish in fast-food emporiums or sold as breaded fish fillets in other outlets after deep-fat frying. No matter how compelling the name or the decoration, it's not for you! These fish do not contain EPA; they contain too much saturated fat, rich in arachidonic acid, and are loaded with salt. They are a great big negative in your quest to conquer inflammation.

Don't ruin good tuna, salmon, trout, or any fish with rich sauces made with mayonnaise or tartar sauce. Learn to use lemon juice, garlic and onions, olive oil, and mushrooms.

Processed Fish

A new technology we call re-formed fish is appearing in our supermarkets. This technology uses fish scraps and scrap fish. By appropriate processing, the scrap is re-formed to look and taste like much more expensive fish such as king crab, lobster, and shrimp. In general this ersatz fish is a good low-fat protein source, but it contains no EPA, although someday, as this diet plan spreads, EPA could be added.

Occasionally it's okay to eat the frozen fish fingers from the supermarket frozen-food section. But learn to read the ingredient list and select those fish that contain the least amount of eggs, salt, and vegetable oil.

Fish: Do's for Arthritis Relief	
Finfish	
High EPA	
Anchovy	Mullet
Dogfish	Sablefish
Eel	Salmon
Herring	Trout
Mackerel	

Fish: Do's for Arthritis Relief

Moderate EPA

Bluefish	Smelt
Carp	Sturgeon
Catfish	Tuna
Sea trout	Whitefish

Low EPA

Bass	Perch
Cod	Pike
Dolphinfish	Plaice
Drum	Pompano
Flounder	Shark
Grouper	Sheepshead
Hake	Sole
Halibut	Swordfish

Crustaceans and Mollusks
High EPA

Conch

Moderate EPA

Oysters

Low EPA

Crab	Mussel
Lobster	Octopus
Shrimp	Scallop
Abalone	Squid
Clam	

5. DO INCLUDE BIRDS

Chicken, turkey, pheasant, guinea fowl, squab, and other birds are all low in fat and excellent sources of protein. Select the breast and the light meat of the leg, but avoid dark meat and don't eat the wings.

Waterfowl is mostly dark meat, but although richer in unsaturated fat, the breast is definitely acceptable. Therefore duck and goose breast are fine. Apply the rule of not eating the skin; if possible, remove it before cooking.

Do use sliced turkey breast sandwiches. The ideal turkey breast is wrapped in skin; simply remove it before or after slicing. Make your sandwiches with Egg Beater mayonnaise. Use lots of lettuce, whole-grain bread, and tomatoes, if your diary tells you they are okay.

Frozen chicken or turkey—even canned is all right. Simply apply the rules of using the breast with skin removed and you're home free.

Barbequed chicken is sometimes prepared before your eyes in glass ovens on a rotisserie. It's okay, but it would be better if the skin were removed first. Remove the skin and stick to the white meat of the breast.

Cooking Birds

Bake, broil, barbeque, or boil for use in salads. If you must fry, use the same rules for fish. Use olive oil and bread with skim milk, egg whites, or Egg Beaters after removing the skin. Fried, breaded chicken with the skin is often too tempting, so remove the skin first!

In making chicken or turkey salad, the major problem is how to avoid mayonnaise if you don't like Egg Beater mayonnaise. This can be accomplished by using plain yogurt and acquiring a taste for the chicken or turkey without adding fat. Salad dressing, especially creamy Italian, works very well.

Take-Out Chicken, Processed-Turkey, etc.

Don't ever eat take-out fried chicken again. Deep-fat frying is a great way to ruin an excellent low-fat, high-quality food.

Don't be deceived by turkey and chicken processed into the form of franks, salami, ham, pastrami, and other well-known don'ts. These products are made using the organs, skin, and other waste materials left after turkey and chicken are processed. They may be all right for active children, but not for you. Don't be deceived; simply avoid them.

Don't use a prebasted turkey at Thanksgiving time. The very name should tell you how it's made. The manufacturers know that most Americans love fat, so they inject fat right into the turkey breast. A regular un-"butterballed" turkey tastes just as good and costs less for the same amount of turkey.

Poultry: Do's for Arthritis Relief

Chicken, including cornish game hen, fryers, broilers, and capons
Chicken roll, light meat only
Canned chicken, light meat only
Turkey, light meat
Turkey roll, light meat only
Duck, breast without skin
Goose, breast without skin
Guinea fowl, breast without skin
Quail, skin removed
Squab, skin removed

---

6. DON'T EAT MOST MEAT

Your objective is to eliminate as much arachidonic acid and saturated fat as possible. In general this means red meat is out.

Don't eat beef, pork, veal, buffalo, and lamb. In fact, if it walked on four legs, it's out.

If something can be worse, organ meats are, and should not even be considered, let alone cooked. Avoid them at all costs.

Processed meats are similarly worse than meat. I know that sounds like double-talk, but it isn't. Processed meat contains about 70% of its calories as saturated fat. It's made from all the organs and by-products; consequently that sausage or hot dog contains stomachs, lungs, livers, kidneys, spleen, and anything I've overlooked.

Processed meat means sausage of any type, franks, bologna, liverwurst, salami, and most other sandwich or luncheon meats. It makes no difference whether the package claims it comes from some exotic animal such as kangaroo, koala, or even birds. Leave it alone.

Occasionally eat rabbit and venison. Rabbit is generally very low in fat. Rabbit thighs and breasts are excellent. Although I do not have analyses of rabbit meat, I believe it might contain some EPA, especially if the animals were fed on grass in a cool climate. It might contain alpha linolenic acid, which we can convert to EPA.

Venison should similarly be fine for an occasional meal. Although rabbit and venison are not regularly eaten in the average household, they are sometimes available in gourmet restaurants and food shops.

Some anthropologists believe that all game of years past did contain EPA or alpha linolenic acid, because game animals ate plant food (leaves and some nuts), which contained them. This could still be the case unless the rabbit and venison are taken from domesticated hutches and herds, then fattened on corn.

What If You're Trapped?

Occasionally you will be trapped. You will find yourself invited to dinner and lo and behold a beautiful roast, chicken livers, steak, or a pâté is put in front of you. Don't panic!

It will do no harm if occasionally you consume a small portion of well-trimmed red meat. Arthur Godfrey had two rules that always worked: Trim off all the fat; then eat only half of what remains.

Don't forget, you've still got to get EPA.

Willpower to trim the fat and reduce the portion will always help. Remember to critique it in your food diary.

Barbara, a person who follows this plan with much success, and uses it in a self-help group, explained to me just how difficult it can be:

"My daughter is graduating from high school and one of the parents had a reception for some other parents in honor of the occasion. The hors d'oeuvres were mostly meat or chicken livers wrapped in bacon. I ate them without thinking and paid the price the next day. My knees and hands swelled and they hurt. I hadn't realized just how effective

---

Meat: Don'ts for Arthritis Relief

Red meats and organ meats (canned, fresh, or smoked)
Beef
Lamb
Pork
Bacon
Ham
Veal
Poultry dark meat
Organ meats from poultry
Processed luncheon meats such as bologna
Frankfurters and sausages
Sandwich spreads from meat
Poultry franks and sausages such as chicken franks and
    turkey franks
Poultry luncheon meats such as chicken or turkey salami,
    pastrami, etc.

this diet was for me until I went off it. I sure have learned my lesson."

This comment illustrates that no matter how well your diet appears to work, the old problem is just waiting to return. Don't let it.

7. DO USE LOTS OF PASTA

Pasta is an excellent way of obtaining both protein and complex carbohydrate. Read the ingredient list to be sure the first ingredient is wheat, spinach (spinach pasta), or corn (corn pasta), and that if eggs appear (preferably they will not), they are far down on the list. Remember, ingredient lists go from maximum to minimum in content, so use them as a means of seeing what you pay for.

With pasta the sauce is king, and that's where this diet can become complex if you don't exercise caution. Proceed carefully.

The best sauce for pasta is a fish, chicken, or clam sauce made with olive oil and absolutely no cream. Sauces generally described as a light clam or fish sauce are superb. These sauces work very well with slivers of chicken or turkey, and green vegetables such as broccoli and parsley; use garlic liberally! Parmesan cheese is desirable for flavor, but it must be used sparingly.

Tomato sauce is the traditional standby for pasta, and tomatoes are in the "nightshade" class of foods. I recommend experimenting with all vegetables, including tomatoes and tomato sauce, because everyone is not affected by these foods. I have encountered many arthritics who can use tomatoes with no problems whatsoever. On the other hand, I have met many who cannot, so you must try for yourself. The following letter, showing the power of a food diary, explains it all.

Dear Dr. Scala,

Thank you for sending me your arthritis diet material. I immediately started to eliminate the don'ts from my diet and am taking EPA . . .

I found when I was in Florida that I was not able to eat grapefruit, as my knees and elbows became sore. I found last summer when our tomatoes were producing a good crop, I was foolish to eat a lot of them. My joints became very sore and when I stopped eating tomatoes the pain went away. I have found that since following your diet, my ankles are not puffy at night as they have been for a long time.

Because Mary, the writer, is 70 years old, this letter brings out two points: It is essential to test certain foods, because what is all right for some is not all right for others. And it states very clearly that you are never too old to improve your life.

Mary's observation that her ankles are not as puffy is consistent with an Air Force doctor who has used a stricter version of this diet. In his words: "I notice within the first week my arthritis complaints disappear and puffiness around the ankles is gone."

So Mary at age 70 is right on target.

Caution: Pasta Sauce

Hopefully, you will have determined by your food diary that tomatoes are fine for you. If so, tomato sauce is the choice for pasta. It is low in fat, low in calories, and nourishing. It can be made from plum tomatoes, regular tomatoes, and tomato paste. Tomato sauce is an excellent vehicle for such vegetables as carrot slices, broccoli, parsley, garlic, onions, and mushrooms. Sautéing of these condiment vegetables should be done in olive oil with added garlic. It can also be converted to a red clam sauce by simply adding canned baby clams.

Don't ever use meat sauce, meat balls, sausage, or any animal fat.

Occasionally pasta needs Parmesan cheese. Use it sparingly. It can be stretched with garlic, parsley, oregano, and other spices and condiments.

8. USE DAIRY PRODUCTS WITH CAUTION

Dairy products cause flare-ups in some arthritics. I know of one woman who cannot even use yogurt. In my opinion, it is not the fat that is responsible, but some other material—possibly the protein or, in technical terms, a "peptide." But names don't matter unless you're a scientist; the point is clear. Test yourself. Use your food diary to identify dairy products you can use and those you cannot use.

Do try nonfat dairy products and dairy products such as cottage cheese and yogurt made from skim or nonfat milk. Milk fat is saturated fat and usually contains arachidonic acid.

Although drinking skim milk, with its bluish cast, is not generally pleasant, it is better than low-fat milk as the following example provides.

Consider a breakfast of Spoon Size Shredded Wheat. This cereal provides 110 calories with 1 gram of fat; that's 9 calories from fat. Nonfat milk has almost no fat calories, therefore the ½ cup of nonfat milk with the cereal contains only 155 calories (45 from milk, 110 from cereal) and 1 gram or 9 calories from fat. That's only 6% of calories from fat—for all practical purposes an insignificant percentage.

Suppose you use low-fat milk. The same cereal—1 ounce with ½ cup low-fat milk—provides about 190 calories, but now with 4 grams of fat (1 from cereal, 3 from milk), which means that 36 of the 190 calories or 19% come from fat. Obviously, this is not the best way to eat your cereal, because our objective is to reduce milk fat to a minimum while keeping the calories from fat to a minimum. But 19% of calories is low fat.

This example with Spoon Size Shredded Wheat was given to show that when you reduce the use of fat-containing foods, you help yourself considerably with very little sacrifice in flavor. For a flavor bonus, include some fruit on the cereal (e.g., 70 to 100 calories from sliced bananas or strawberries), adding more fiber, flavor, and reducing the percentage of calories from fat to 3.5% for the skim milk and only 12.4% for the low-fat milk, respectively. You can't lose by adding fruit.

A better cereal would be oatmeal. Mother's Rolled Oats provides excellent fiber and about the same calories as the Spoon Size Shredded Wheat, so the same example would apply; the fruit of choice would be raisins added during cooking, topped with sliced bananas for serving.

I get many recipes that people devise to help them get around sensitive foods. A number of people who like oatmeal but cannot use even skim milk use apricot nectar in place of milk. My family tried it and we all like it. Other people use the nondairy creamers that are available.

Cottage cheese with 1% fat is fine. Occasionally low-fat mozzarella is acceptable, but it should be used sparingly. All other cheese, except ricotta and Parmesan sparingly on pasta, are *Don'ts* on this diet.

Yogurt made from skim milk or from nonfat dry milk is excellent. It is especially good if fruit is included. However, yogurt made from whole milk should not be used.

Ricotta cheese, if used in a meal such as stuffed shells or stuffed manicotti is okay if the meal also contains generous servings of vegetables and the pasta portion is small. Ricotta cheese can be mixed with cottage cheese, parsley, broccoli and, of all things, unprocessed bran, and carbohydrate calories can be added by an appropriate sauce. Careful planning is required to reduce the calories from fat to an absolute minimum, however—no more than 15% of calories.

Sherbet can be used as often as you wish for dessert. All

flavors are fine and they are especially nutritious when topped with fruit.

Pudding made with skim milk is another acceptable dessert. Let's do some arithmetic: ½ cup butterscotch pudding made from a mix with low-fat milk contains 4.7 grams of fat; that's 42 calories from fat out of a total of 171 calories (most from carbohydrate), or only 25% of its calories from fat. Add some fruit such as bananas and you've reduced the fat to less than 20% of calories. Use skim milk and the pudding is great!

Searching will produce all kinds of dessert recipes that make use of skim milk, cottage and ricotta cheese and are low in fat. Just remember to keep the fat calories as low as possible and always less than 25% of total calories. By topping with fruit, you introduce more carbohydrate, reducing the fat-calorie percentage, and introduce dietary fiber.

A Dairy Wasteland

Don't eat any high-fat dairy products. Once you get past the nonfat dairy products made with skim milk (such as cottage cheese or yogurt), it becomes a wasteland of *Don'ts*. That includes ice cream, cheese, and most other dairy products.

Once in a While

Occasionally have ice milk for dessert and top with fruit.

Occasionally you can eat a vegetarian pizza with skim milk mozzarella cheese, lots of garlic, onions, green peppers, and olives. Cook on a "Pizza Brick" to help reduce the oil content of the final dish.

9. DON'T USE WHOLE EGGS

Egg white is fine wherever required (ie, recipes, breading mix, etc) The egg yolk is the problem; don't eat it except under the circumstances described as "occasionally."

Dairy Product Do's for Arthritis Relief

Cheese

Cottage cheese (low-fat or skim milk)

Mozzarella (skim milk)—limited intake

Parmesan (grated)—sparingly

Ricotta (skim milk)

Milk

Skim

Skim protein fortified

Skim made from dry milk

Yogurt

Skim milk yogurt

Dairy Desserts

Ice milk—occasionally

Sherbet

Dairy Product Don'ts for Arthritis Relief

Whole milk

Lowfat (2% fat) milk

Homogenized milk

Evaporated and condensed milk

Buttermilk

Goat milk

Soybean milk

Yogurt from whole milk

Cheese from whole milk

Egg yolks

Butter

Do use egg substitutes whenever possible. Such products as Egg Beaters are excellent for recipes that use the whole egg, such as scrambled eggs, omelets, and French toast.

Check Your Food Diary

Occasionally use egg yolks in recipes in which there are at least four servings for every egg yolk. That is the equivalent of about ¼ egg.

Some dietary experimentalists have informed me that by testing with a food diary they can eat an egg occasionally. But, if they don't put at least one day in between the eggs, they start to see swelling and the flare-up. Trial and error is the key to success along with a well-used food diary.

Don't use whole eggs for cooking unless the yolk is absolutely necessary and the final product (e.g., a cake) will be divided into many pieces.

10. DO EAT GENEROUS AMOUNTS OF CEREALS AND GRAINS

Do eat lots of cereals and grains. You can't use too much, no matter how hard you try. Breakfast cereals are excellent, especially those made from whole grain. The objective of eating cereals is to obtain dietary fiber, especially soluble dietary fiber such as gums and saponins as are found in oatmeal. Because the American way is to use prepared food, however, learn what to look for in packaged cereal ingredient lists.

The first ingredient should be the substance of the cereal; for example, oats, corn bran, wheat.

Preferably the cereal will not contain either sugar or corn syrup, but if it contains one, it is still okay.

There should be a listing that shows "Dietary Fiber" per serving. On this plan you should select cereals that provide at least 4 grams of fiber and preferably more, up to 9 grams.

Chapter 7 lists cereals that provide adequate dietary fiber without a lot of sugar.

Eat breakfast cereals with skim milk and fruit, and use sugar sparingly; try brown sugar, honey, or maple syrup instead of granulated sugar.

Many Americans think of cereals and grains only as something to eat for breakfast. But these excellent sources of fiber, complex carbohydrate, and protein also include the following:

Barley, especially pearled barley.

Corn, from corn off the cob to cornmeal. Corn pasta is available for those who have severe allergies to wheat. It requires special cooking but is a fine way to add more vegetables to your diet.

Rice, excellent in carbohydrate, fiber, and with appropriate accompaniments, protein. Rice has everything going for it and nothing against it. Rice comes in many forms, including long grain, wild, and polished.

Wheat, or Wheat Germ, in the form of cooked cracked wheat (a side dish such as rice or potatoes). Add a sauce that is low in fat or mix the wheat with rice.

Whole-grain Bread. Use spreads such as olive oil, peanut, or sesame oil. Peanut butter or almond butter unsalted are also acceptable.

Don't Go Wrong

Don't use homogenized or whole milk on breakfast cereals. Learn to do without sugar, or with a small amount.

Occasionally take a break from the standard. Remember, this is a lifelong commitment; therefore try different foods such as grits, barley, and so on. Switch around and let variety work for you. Cereals and grains can only help and never hurt in your search for relief, so use them generously.

Grain and Grain Products: Do's for Arthritis Relief

Breads and Rolls

Bagel	Italian
Biscuits (nonbuttermilk)	Matzo
Brown bread	Mixed grain
Brown bread with raisins	Raisin
Cracked wheat	Rye (all types)
French	Sourdough
Fresh horizons white or	Wheat
wheat	Wheatberry
Hollywood dark and light	White (low sodium)
Honey wheatberry	

Crackers

Melba toast	RyeKrisp
Rice wafer	Triscuits
Rusk	Zwieback

Dinner Rolls

Brown and serve	Wheat
French	White, hard
Raisin	Whole wheat
Rye, hard	

Muffins

English muffins (plain and	Whole wheat
sourdough)	Bran

Noodles

Asian dry	Soba
Rice	Enriched
Saimin	

Grain and Grain Products: Do's for Arthritis Relief

Pancakes

Most pancakes are made from mixes. Unprocessed bran can be added to the batter to increase their dietary fiber. Egg Beaters can replace eggs in the mix.

Plain	Cornmeal
Buttermilk	Soy
Buckwheat	

Waffles

Waffles are generally higher in fat than pancakes. Unprocessed bran can be added to the batter; Egg Beaters can replace eggs.

Cooked Cereals

Barley	Oatmeal
Buckwheat	Ralston
Cream of wheat	Whole wheat

Cold (Ready to Eat) Cereals

All bran (all brands including extra fiber)	Oat bran
	Wheat bran
40% Bran flakes (all brands)	Wheaties
Bran buds	Most
Raisin bran	Nutri-grain wheat and raisins
Shredded wheat	
Corn bran	

---

11. DO INCLUDE LOTS OF VEGETABLES

If I have things my way, you will learn that with the exception of breakfast, you should eat a vegetable or two with each meal, together with a green salad. Breakfast should always include fruit. The rewards are more than worth the effort and investment.

There is no end to the variety of vegetables in this world and no end to their varied colors and tastes. They all provide various levels of dietary fiber, are generally good sources of potassium, the B vitamins, and vitamin C. *Don't* forget, though, that the "nightshade vegetables" present a problem to some people.

The best way to prepare vegetables is to steam them lightly so they are still crunchy. Stir-frying is excellent, but only if you use olive oil or Puritan oil. Soybean oil or peanut oil are okay, but they are second best, and corn oil is out.

Frozen vegetables are fine. They retain their nutrients, fiber, and their taste, contrary to popular opinion—or should I say misconception. They offer more nutrients than "fresh" counterparts, even if they have been sitting in a supermarket or on a truck for a few days or even weeks.

Canned vegetables are not as good as frozen because they often contain too much salt and sometimes too much sugar. Canned vegetables contain about as much fiber as their frozen or fresh counterparts. If there are no alternatives to canned vegetables, then use them, but only as an alternate to fresh or frozen in that order.

BEANS

Do remember beans deserve a special place in your diet. A serving of kidney beans of 120 calories provides about 25% as protein, 85% as carbohydrate, and no fat. Each 3½-ounce serving provides 5 grams of dietary fiber. Therefore a meal of beans, rice, a salad, and another vegetable is by any standards, excellent.

Salad possibilities with beans are also appealing—as long as olive oil or Puritan oil is used in the dressing.

For years people have called beans the "musical fruit." This is a polite reference to the flatulence, the gas that develops when people eat beans for a meal. Beans frequently contain factors in the fiber fraction that cause flatulence, but this passes as the body acclimates to them, especially if they are used in moderation.

Canned beans are fine; just select ones that contain no pork or other animal products. Baked beans made with molasses or other nonanimal fat components are excellent. One more reminder to avoid canned beans with fat added, because a great food is diminished in quality; for this diet, destroyed.

Garlic, Onions, Chives, Shallots, etc.

Do use garlic and onions.

Perhaps only people in Gilroy, California, the "garlic capital" sit down to fried garlic and sautéed onions, but if more people did, they would be doing themselves a favor. These two foods contain materials that help the prostaglandins perform their functions.

In fact, research has shown that natural materials in garlic and onions can actually act as prostaglandins to some extent. You simply can't use too much garlic, onions, and other condiments such as shallots and leeks. You must, however, take into account your friends, next of kin, loved ones, business associates, and anyone else who might come in contact with your breath and body odor.

Cooking Vegetables

Cooking vegetables is just about as simple or as elaborate as you want it to be. Steam until crisp, but cooked; boil if you must or stir-fry in olive oil; add garlic to taste.

Don't cook vegetables in corn oil, butter, animal fat, or other fatty materials. Olive oil is the choice for cooking oil.

Occasionally try something really new. There is such a variety of vegetables available; take time to test all of them. You can't explore the variety in a lifetime: jicama, Jerusalem artichoke, water chestnuts, and salsify, to name but a few.

Caution: Vegetables, Grains, and Cereals

Occasionally people are sensitive, even allergic, to such foods as corn, wheat, and others. Use your food diary as the means of identifying food sensitivity.

Vegetables: Do's for Arthritis Relief	
Alfalfa sprouts	Cauliflower
Artichokes	Celeriac root
Asparagus	Celery
Avocado	Chard
Bamboo shoots	Chicory
Beans (canned with molasses or brown sugar)	Chives
Beans, white cooked	Collard greens
Beets	Corn, white or yellow
Beet greens	Cowpeas
Black-eyed peas	Cucumber
Broccoli	Dandelion greens
Brussel sprouts	Eggplants
Butter beans	Endive
Cabbage	Fennel
Carrots	Garbanzo beans (chick-peas)

Vegetables: Do's for Arthritis Relief

Ginger root
Green beans (Italian and snap)
Hominy
Jerusalem artichoke
Kale
Kidney beans, red
Kohlrabi
Leeks
Lentils
Lettuce
Lima beans
Mung bean sprouts
Mushrooms
Mustard greens
Mustard spinach
Okra
Onions
Parsley
Peas
Pepper, bell
Pimentos
Potato, white (caution)

Pumpkin
Purslane
Radishes, red
Rhubarb
Scallions
Shallots
Snow peas
Spinach
Squash (acorn, butternut, hubbard, zucchini, summer, and winter)
Sweet potato
Tomato (caution)
Turnip
Turnip greens
Water chestnuts
Watercress
Wax beans
Winged beans
Yams
Yambeans
Yautia

12. DO ADD FRUIT

Do become a fanatic for fruit consumption. You can never eat too much fruit! The variety is enormous, and it's all great for you. Fruit, for all practical purposes, has no fat, it's high in soluble fiber that is excellent for arthritis—and the fiber moderates the simple sugars of fruit so they provide us with lots of energy without large changes in blood sugar.

I want you to eat fruit as dessert, as snacks, as a garnish for cereal. Fruit provides bulk to a meal and can make a light meal more filling. For example, a medium banana, which delivers 100 calories, contains no fat, little protein, and about 25 grams of carbohydrate. Bananas are filling, they seem to contain fat but don't, are pleasant to eat, and provide dietary fiber, vitamins, and minerals. Bananas are great by themselves, on cereal, in low-fat yogurt, as a flaming dessert, or as a simple snack.

Caution: Dried Fruit

Dried fruits by themselves are fine. But sometimes they are treated with sulfite to help preservation. Sulfite can be detrimental to people with inflammatory problems, especially asthmatics. If you ever see it on an ingredient list or find it was used in processing, don't purchase the product. Vote with your pocketbook to eliminate unwanted additives and processing aids; industry will hear you.

Do: Other Fruits

"An apple a day," a saying, that originated over 800 years ago in England, was good advice then, but is better advice today. Apples provide dietary fiber, minerals, vitamins, and satisfaction. And don't stop with apples; think peach, orange, pear, citrus fruits, banana, blueberries, blackberries, strawberries, watermelon, cantaloupe, melon of any kind, and any other fruit or berry you can think of. Try them all and, unless your food diary says otherwise, they are good for you.

Canned fruit is generally canned in sugar syrup, which should be drained before use. If you can get fruit canned in its own juices, great; similarly for frozen fruit or fruit mixes. Simply read the ingredient list and if it's got sugar or corn syrup, don't use it regularly.

Fruit Juice in Disguise

Fruit juices are okay if they are the whole juice. For example, fresh-squeezed orange juice or whole frozen orange juice is fine. So is apple, pear, apricot, prune, guava, pineapple, strawberry, even banana, and others.

Don't use fruit juice unless it's a natural juice of the whole fruit. Natural juices are usually cloudy because they contain the fiber and some starches. Don't use clarified juice. Fruit juice isn't always what you think; for example, read the ingredient list on a can of Hawaiian Punch. You will see that it's about 10% juice and the remainder is various forms of sugar and flavors.

Caution: Fruit

There are occasionally fruits that will cause a reaction. Either some material in the fruit or other food resembles the materials that elicit the inflammatory response or they interact with the metabolic pathways that produce the moderators such as EPA. Perhaps it's a form of allergy, which some doctors describe as a sensitivity.

I wish I could be more definitive in my caution. You must experiment through the use of your food diary. Science simply doesn't have the answer and there are no simple tests that are valid. A thorough examination of all the medical literature has convinced me that personal experience is the best guide. And the value of fruit is so important that to rule out any class of fruit categorically would be wrong.

Suspect fruits include grapefruit, pineapple, and a few berries such as blueberries and tomatoes—yes, tomatoes are berries.

Fruits and Whole Juices: Do's for Arthritis Relief	
Acerola	Lemon
Amaranth	Loganberries
Apples (all types)	Loquats
Applesauce, unsweetened	Lychees
Apricots	Mangos
Bananas	Mulberries
Blackberries	Nectarines
Blueberries	Oranges (all types)
Boysenberries	Papaya
Canteloupe	Passionfruit
Carambola	Peaches
Casaba melon	Pears
Cherries	Persimmons
Cranberries	Pineapple
Currants (all types)	Plantain
Dates (dried)	Plum
Elderberries	Pomegranates
Figs (all types)	Pricklypears
Gooseberries	Prunes
Grapefruit	Raspberries
Grapes (all types)	Sapodilla
Guava	Strawberries
Honeydew melon	Tangelos
Jackfruit	Tangerines
Kiwifruit	Watermelon
Kumquats	

Nuts

Caution. Nuts, like fruit, must be subjected to testing. In general they contain a great deal of fat and too often they are heavily salted. If the salt isn't enough, artificial "smoke" flavor is often added. Read the ingredient list!

I recommend nuts as the "fruit" of a tree—walnuts, cashews, almonds, pecans, hazelnuts, pine nuts, and so on.

Remember, nuts contain a lot of calories.

When nuts are used in recipes their fat is generally diluted and they present a lesser concern.

Rated for Arthritis Relief
Almonds (fair) Cashews (good) Chestnuts (excellent) Litchi nuts (excellent) Soybean nuts (good) Walnuts (good, alpha linolenic acid) Pine nuts (fair)

13. DO TAKE SUPPLEMENTS

There are nineteen vitamins and minerals required to maintain a good nutritional foundation for your health. If you follow this diet plan, you will on average do well. But I believe in leaving nothing to chance in a world that has everything available. Therefore select a supplement that has the following: the RDA for all the vitamins and minerals in two to four tablets daily. The most common, Shaklee Vita-Lea, provides all the nutrients except calcium and magnesium, which it provides at about 60% RDA in two tablets. It is an excellent supplement model; take at least one tablet per day and get at least one-half the RDA in everything except calcium and magnesium. Calcium and magnesium are simply too bulky for a complete single multivitamin-multimineral supplement. They can be obtained from another supplement called "calcium and magnesium."

Do add a calcium supplement. If you take one Vita-Lea tablet each day, you should still obtain the equivalent of 3½ glasses of milk. For each glass of nonfat milk or nonfat yogurt you skip or omit, use a calcium supplement of from 225 to 300 milligrams.

Calcium is found in many dark green vegetables such as broccoli and spinach. So if you take two or three calcium tablets containing about 250 milligrams of calcium, you will do fine. Take only one tablet of no greater than 300 milligrams with a meal. And be sure you always take your calcium supplement at mealtime, because calcium requires other food components such as carbohydrate for efficient absorption.

Do use EPA-eicosapentaenoic acid. I want you to use supplemental EPA each day in addition to eating blue-skinned fish to assure you get at least 1 gram of dietary EPA. Most EPA supplements contain 180 milligrams of EPA in each capsule; therefore you should take six capsules daily as your insurance. To be certain, however, divide 1,000 by the number of milligrams of EPA in each capsule to obtain your daily number of capsules. For example, you would require three 360 milligram capsules, four 260 milligram capsules, or six 180 milligram capsules.

One thing you're sure to notice is that some EPA capsules have a "fishy" aftertaste and even a gaseous rebound. This usually passes after you've used them for a week or two. This fish rebound, as I call it, can also be reduced by taking the capsules with a meal or at bedtime when the stomach is quiet.

Do eat fiber supplements. I have urged lots of fruit, vegetables, grains, and other sources of dietary fiber on you. But even then I find many people don't get enough fiber. There are several means available to supplement with fiber.

Fiber wafers make an excellent snack. Be sure the label explains how much fiber. It should balance out to about 5 grams fiber per 100 calories. Always drink lots of water with it.

Vegetable fiber supplement—the most common fiber supplement is Metamucil or copies of Metamucil. Be sure you mix with adequate water.

Unbalanced Supplements

Don't use unbalanced supplements. There are many supplements on the market, some of which purport to have incredible properties. These can be identified by having none to 100% of the RDA of one or two components; then, 1,000% or 500% in others and possibly 10% or less of others. Simply don't use them.

14. CAUTION: BEVERAGES

Do drink lots of water; you should consume four to eight glasses of water daily. Much of our water is consumed as other beverages, but if you resolve to drink at least four glasses of actual water, you will be helping to make your dietary fiber even more effective. And, water will help your body eliminate unwanted metabolic by-products. That's sophisticated talk for waste materials.

Mineral water is an excellent beverage; you can't drink too much. Seek out one with lots of magnesium.

Do limit coffee intake and other caffeine-containing beverages. The equivalent of two cups of coffee daily is sufficient caffeine without being excessive. Two cups is about 150 to 200 milligrams of caffeine. Because decaffeinated coffee contains no caffeine, it doesn't matter.

Tea contains about 35 milligrams of caffeine per cup, so you can have four to six cups of tea without reaching your upper limit. An additional benefit of tea is it is gentle on the stomach. Tea actually promotes stomach emptying and avoids an acid rebound. This is an advantage if you are using aspirin or one of the aspirin derivatives for medication. Indeed, in my opinion, the beverage of choice for ulcer sufferers (often arthritics) is tea. And the best tea is standard black tea, such as Lipton's.

In contrast to tea, coffee elicits an acid rebound. That

means that when you drink coffee on an empty stomach, your stomach produces an excessive amount of acid and overshoots its mark, creating an excessively acidic condition. Although this is not inherently bad because we normally don't drink coffee on an empty stomach, it doesn't help if you are using medication such as aspirin or an aspirin derivative, which already has an effect on the stomach.

Occasionally enjoy soft drinks. But remember that if they are not artificially sweetened (diet drinks), they contain about 7 teaspoons of sugar and many also contain about 35 milligrams of caffeine per 8 ounces. Choose from the wide variety of diet, caffeine-free soft drinks available today.

Caution: Alcoholic Beverages

Wine can turn a good meal into a superb dining experience. Similarly a cocktail can make an ordinary predinner discussion an elegant encounter. Moderation is the key word.

Although alcohol has never been proven to alter the course of inflammation, it does interact with some medication. In fact, it usually creates the potential for problems.

Excessive alcohol interferes with metabolism—specifically fat metabolism, and indirectly that is what this dietary plan is all about. Indeed, a cocktail, a glass of wine with dinner, a glass of beer is no problem. It only becomes a problem when excess prevails, so use caution and good judgment.

CHAPTER
11 Menu Planning

This chapter translates the *Do's* and *Don'ts* into suggestions for breakfast, lunch, dinner, and snacks. The menu plans are based on interviews with people who have succeeded, such as a 35-year-old mother, a woman of 45 whose children are grown, a retired couple, and others, including a teenage girl with an entire life ahead of her. My hope is that you will see yourself or a loved one here and find ideas that fit your taste and lifestyle.

BREAKFAST: GETTING STARTED

This is the most important meal of the day, no matter how old you are, what you do in life, and where you do it. Breakfast will influence how you will feel all day (or night if you work nights), so approach it with the respect it deserves.

Our objective at breakfast is to obtain calories in the form of complex carbohydrates containing some dietary fiber. Protein, which is necessary for all bodily processes, also helps us maintain constant blood sugar, which helps keep our moods even.

Morning is also an ideal time to take general supplements, especially a multivitamin and mineral, some calcium, and EPA. It is also an excellent time to exercise (see Chapter 14).

BREAKFAST FOODS

Fruit is ideal at breakfast; it can be put on cereal, eaten alone, or mixed in a blender to make a "shake" for people in a hurry. There is no limit to breakfast fruit, but some are typical:

Grapefruit—the old favorite—a half grapefruit, sectioned, part of a fruit compote, baked or microwaved with some honey or brown sugar on top.

Oranges sliced or in a compote.

Kiwi fruit, halved and spooned out with a grapefruit spoon, almost like ice cream.

Papaya scooped or sliced like a melon.

Melon of any type, including cantaloupe, honeydew, crenshaw, Spanish, watermelon, and several others.

Strawberries sliced with yogurt, served plain, or as toppings for cereal.

Bananas are fine alone, but are excellent sliced on cereal. Their texture adds to the enjoyment of any cereal. They are not high in calories, contain no fat (contrary to popular belief), and are an excellent source of potassium.

Berries—raspberries, blueberries, and blackberries, to name a few—are delicious by themselves, on cereal, or with yogurt.

Mangoes are superb and becoming more readily available. They are tricky to eat—slice in half (lengthwise) and turn inside out, and slice off in chunks. The first one is difficult, but it gets easier.

Prunes in syrup or on cereal are also excellent to get things moving.

Fiber is one of the most important nutritional objectives of breakfast, and fruit can make a significant contribution. For example, most typical fruit servings supply from 1.5 to 5 grams of dietary fiber (5 grams is about 20% of our daily need), and fruit fiber is excellent because much of it falls into the soluble category that helps remove waste materials from the system.

FRUIT JUICE

Nothing is so overrated nutritionally and enjoyed by so many people. We all like a glass of juice in the morning, so let's all make a vow to drink genuine fruit juice. Frozen is fine; canned is fine. Read the ingredient list and ask some questions. Does it contain the juice of real fruit? If so, great. Does it contain sugar or corn syrup? If so, bad! Does it contain salt as one of the top three ingredients? If so, avoid it!

Fresh squeezed is the best. Remember, real juice is usually cloudy and often tastes somewhat bland. Orange juice, apple juice, tomato juice (V-8 also), prune juice, papaya juice, grapefruit juice, or pineapple juice should contain pulp and not be clear. And they're all excellent.

CEREAL

Conduct a test. Take a piece of cereal and place it on your tongue with a lot of saliva. Swish it around for a few minutes. Is any significant residue left? If not, don't bother to eat it because it's probably mostly sugar; if it leaves a good residue, it contains what you're after in a good cereal—fiber.

Conduct a reading test. Does the ingredient list contain sugar or corn syrup before some real cereal—like corn? Is the sugar or corn syrup or both one of the first three ingredients? If so, don't use it!

Although I have not tested each cereal in this way, I have

prepared a list (Chapter 7) for you, which provides at least 3 grams of dietary fiber in a standard 1-ounce serving. Following is an abbreviated approach:

Cooked cereals: Oat as oatmeal either regular or instant, Ralston, Wheatena, or Cream of Wheat.

Bran cereals: First the 100% Bran type (All-Bran, Corn Bran, etc.).

Second, the modified bran (40% Bran Flakes) such as Kellogg's Bran Flakes, raisin bran, Cracklin' Bran, Most, and so on.

Third are the "grain" cereals, which imply that they are more "natural." In general, they contain a reasonable amount of fiber and include enticing names such as Heartland, Nutri-Grain, 100% Natural, and so on.

Ingredient lists: The ingredient list has the ingredients in descending order of content. First should be the major ingredient, such as wheat bran or corn bran, and so on. Then, it will usually contain some sugar or salt, and possibly raisins. If it contains sugar and corn syrup solids, that's camouflage for not having to put sugar first—don't purchase it.

Nutritional label: If the serving size is reasonable (1 ounce, ⅓ to 1 cup, etc.), the cereal should deliver at least 3.5 grams of dietary fiber and preferably at least 5 grams of dietary fiber up to 9 for All-Bran. Please don't settle for less than 3.5 unless it's either oatmeal or cooked Ralston.

Serving: Always use skim milk with as little sugar as possible and as much fruit as you like. Berries and bananas are especially good for convenience and the textural sensation they impart to the eating quality.

I have discussed methods of preparing cereal with many people and nothing surprises me. Oatmeal with apricot nectar was suggested by a woman who cannot use milk; I've tried it and it is excellent.

EGGS VERSUS EGG BEATERS

You've made a commitment to health, but eggs may test your resolve. They do not fit directly into this diet. So use some of the many egg substitutes that are available.

But you can't rely on all egg substitutes, because some of them contain more fat than eggs. My preference is Egg Beaters or Scramblers. There are others, and you must read the nutritional label to be sure they are an improvement over eggs.

Egg Beaters permit you to have scrambled eggs and omelets, which should include vegetables—especially zucchini, mushrooms, onions, chives, broccoli, spinach (precooked), and wheat germ. I have served nutritionists mushroom, onion, and garlic omelets made from Egg Beaters and not one could tell that I didn't use eggs!

The addition of 1 ounce of skim-milk mozzarella cheese will add texture to the omelet. However, it is better to learn to eat strictly vegetarian omelets without cheese.

PANCAKES, WAFFLES, AND FRENCH TOAST

Pancakes and waffles can be made with the addition of unprocessed bran to add fiber, skim milk, Egg Beaters for eggs, and olive oil for shortening. The mix used should emphasize wheat or buckwheat flour as much as possible. Aunt Jemima mixes are my favorites and they work fine with Egg Beaters.

Once the batter is prepared, spoon it onto the griddle and add sliced or diced fruit on top—especially berries (blueberries, raspberries, strawberries), but sliced peaches, apples, and bananas work equally well. Waffles can use fruit as well, but it must be added to the batter. It is usually best to chop the fruit into small pieces so it blends well with the batter.

French toast made with slightly dry sourdough bread soaked in an Egg Beater batter, using skim milk with some mild spice such as nutmeg or cinnamon is excellent.

Topping for pancakes, waffles, and French toast should not include butter; the American classic, maple syrup, is excellent, but so is blueberry or boysenberry syrup or some other natural syrup. Avoid the "glop" made from corn syrup, butter, and artificial flavor.

BRAN MUFFINS

In Chapter 12, "Basic Recipes," I have included the recipe for bran muffins. These muffins provide dietary fiber and have a very unusual feature—the batter keeps for six weeks in the refrigerator. That is correct; you make the batter once every six weeks and it takes no more time to prepare them than to prepare most breakfast foods. Bran muffins are best warm, but they are also satisfying cold.

OTHER POSSIBILITIES FOR BREAKFAST

There is no limit to breakfast; for example, it can be a salad, fish, chicken—anything from the *Do* list. However, breakfast should always provide some fiber, protein, and not much fat. An excellent alternative is a "meal" substitute, which is best made from soy protein and mixed with either skim milk or juice. These are usually marketed as protein supplements or meal substitutes. Use the ingredient list as your guide.

SUPPLEMENTS

Breakfast is the best time to take your multivitamin and mineral supplement. It is also an excellent time to take EPA supplements and supplemental fiber if you do not eat a high-fiber breakfast and a daily diet rich in fish. Take high-fiber snacks during the day or a soluble fiber supplement in the evening.

Calcium supplements should be taken with meals.

"COFFEE BREAK"

An American tradition; indeed most countries have time out for a mid-morning break. In the United States it is usually coffee and some type of snack.

Coffee is okay, tea is better, and juice better yet. But, more important is the snack taken with the coffee (or other beverage). There should be no need for a snack, but that doesn't deter most people, so choose one that provides fiber and complex carbohydrate. If that sounds like fruit, it is! Don't eat doughnuts or sweet rolls; they elevate blood sugar only to let you down later. If you must eat something, make it a bran muffin. Remember, 18% of arthritics suffer from anxiety and depression—don't make it worse with bad snacking habits.

LUNCH

Lunch is often the main meal of the day and it varies according to activity. The executive conducts business over lunch in a restaurant or cafeteria; the homemaker often eats alone—not infrequently while watching a TV soap opera; the working person might "brown bag" a lunch or eat with friends in the company cafeteria. Whatever the circumstances, lunch should accomplish several objectives.

EPA is a nutrient objective that can be obtained from fish (Chapter 4) or as a supplement. Fish can be eaten as a tuna salad or sandwich, a nicely grilled swordfish steak, or can even be smoked trout. It must, by necessity, vary with the circumstances, both lifestyle and economic. With a little imagination fish can be eaten almost every day at lunch. With a little enthusiasm, some imagination, and willpower, lunch can get the bad fat out and the good EPA in.

Protein is always one major objective; indeed, it is often the luncheon feature, especially in a restaurant. The protein can be obtained or enhanced as a garnish on pasta, the clams in a clam sauce, or shredded chicken over rice in a Chinese dish. There is no end to the variety.

Complex carbohydrate is important, especially the complex carbohydrate that comes so elegantly packaged by nature in rice, beans, vegetables, fruit, grains, cereals, and breads. This carbohydrate will provide the energy to carry you for the rest of the day and into the evening.

Dietary fiber, which is obtained with complex carbohydrate—especially in the grains and fruit—is important.

Green leafy vegetables should, whenever possible, be part of every lunch. This is often obtained by the traditional green salad, which can consist of lettuce, spinach, watercress, sprouts, cabbage, and any other leafy vegetable. If you don't have a problem with them, tomatoes are excellent; if they are a problem, cucumbers and zucchini make good substitutes.

AFTERNOON SNACKS

Snacking has become an American pastime. Therefore if you can't fight it, you might as well join it. Snacks usually consist of carbohydrates of the wrong kind—empty calorie sugar—so think of those that would be healthy.

Popcorn is excellent, bran muffins, vegetable sticks, and fruit are all snacks that help you get a little closer to the objectives of this way of life you've chosen.

Tea is the best beverage. If you take soft drinks, use the low-calorie type; remember, the nondiet type contains about 10 teaspoons of sugar per 12-ounce can. Avoid soft drinks if you can.

DINNER

Traditionally dinner is the family gathering time, even in today's fast-paced world in which most people eat at least one and often two meals away from home. It is a chance to talk over the adventures and events of the day, to congratulate each other for a day well spent, and to search for solutions to the problems of today that will make a better day tomorrow.

Such an important gathering must be an enjoyable event, and the menu selected should enhance the fellowship. Our commitment can be shared by everyone and they will be better for the experience. This plan is low in fat, low in cholesterol, and rich in those things that prevent heart disease and reduce the risk of cancer. Further, the eating habits it will instill in children can only help them throughout life. Therefore plan menus that everyone can enjoy.

Dinner is your final opportunity of the day to get EPA from food and not as a supplement. But it is imperative that it not be one-sided—that it be appealing.

EPA is the major objective, but a secondary objective is to keep saturated fat to a minimum and polyunsaturated fat to a reasonable level. Thus the protein choice is important.

Main entrées for dinner can be as elaborate as you wish to make them. Trout stuffed with mushrooms, bread, onions, and scallions sautéed in olive oil laced with garlic is one of our favorites (Chapter 12). But just as good is a piece of broiled frozen swordfish or a tuna salad (Chapter 12) without mayonnaise or with Egg Beater mayonnaise. If it's not fish, it can be as elaborate as pheasant, duck, guinea fowl, or simply breaded, skinned chicken (eat only the breast) sautéed in olive oil with a touch of garlic.

Don't overlook pasta, especially with a light sauce, including chicken, clams, or some other high-protein source. Pasta is always excellent.

Dinner should always include a good source of complex carbohydrate, such as rice, potato, Jerusalem artichoke, squash, carrots, wheat, barley, or millet; and there are others. Pasta can be the major part of the meal, including both protein and carbohydrate.

No dinner is complete without green vegetables such as string beans, asparagus, broccoli, spinach, turnip greens, or other variations. Finally, a green salad should accompany the menu; the carrot and cabbage salad in Chapter 12 is excellent for this program, and everyone likes it.

Dessert has a rich history in our tradition. It has always been the children's reward associated with clearing the plate. By the time we're adults, it's habit—something we expect. Nutritionally it often provided calcium as cheese or a fermented milk product, but that's history.

Many desserts can be made or purchased that are completely acceptable on this plan. Fruit is the most natural, obviously acceptable, and excellent for this plan. In Chapter 12 I have included a basic apple cake, and a few others.

You are trying to avoid butter and egg yolks, although in most recipes these components are diluted over many servings. There are basic recipes that can include margarine, Egg Beaters, and olive oil. And you're home free.

TEN DAYS—TEN MENUS

The following menus were created by people who are gaining control of their arthritis. With these meals—and variations that you can create using Part I of this book and following the *Do's* and *Don'ts* of Chapter 10—you can begin to feel better, too.

DAY 1

A mother with arthritis who prepares food for the entire family. They pull together with her and are better and healthier for the commitment.

BREAKFAST:
- Pancakes made with Aunt Jemima's Buckwhat Pancake and Waffle Mix and skim milk, Egg Beaters, olive oil, and ½ cup unprocessed bran; she adds sliced apples to each pancake immediately after pouring the batter on the griddle.
- Maple syrup—the real kind
- Orange juice, coffee with nondairy creamer
- Bran muffins

LUNCH:
- Barbeque chicken. Charcoal barbequed breasts and legs with the skin removed, using barbeque sauce. For other members of the family, skin was left on while barbequing.
- Three-bean salad, using green, waxed, and kidney beans marinated in Wish-Bone Italian Dressing with onions, crushed garlic clove, and oregano.
- Salad made with lettuce, shaved carrots, sliced zucchini, and green peppers.
- Steamed asparagus
- Fruit salad made with apples, strawberries, melon, and diced pineapple
- Beer (one glass)
- Coffee

DINNER:
- Broiled salmon—pink, juicy, and slightly browned
- Long-grain rice with parsley and shallots
- Sliced zucchini sautéed in olive oil with mushrooms and onions
- Tuna salad sandwich for son who wouldn't eat salmon
- Apple pie

SUPPLEMENTS:
- Calcium: Three
- Vita-Lea: One
- EPA: None
- A fiber supplement

DAY 2

A 33-year-old nonworking mother of children aged 11 and 8. She developed arthritis at age 32. She successfully prepares the same meals for everyone.

BREAKFAST:
- Oatmeal with raisins; she uses skim milk and sugar on her oatmeal. Her husband and children use low-fat milk on theirs.
- Bran muffin with coffee

MID-MORNING:
- Hot tea with an apple

LUNCH:
- Tuna chunks with olive oil and lemon juice mixed with chopped celery, served over a half avocado on top of a lettuce leaf
- Sourdough bread

- Iced tea
- Melon balls topped with strawberry yogurt
- Coffee or tea with oatmeal cookies

DINNER:
- Spinach spaghetti with tomato sauce. The sauce contained shaved carrots, sliced mushrooms (sautéed in olive oil with garlic), onions, oregano, and basil. Sauce was simmered for 4 hours.
- Lettuce and tomato salad with sliced red peppers, zucchini, tomatoes, and asparagus chunks; Wish-Bone Caesar Salad Dressing
- Strawberries over pound cake topped with strawberry yogurt
- Hot tea

SUPPLEMENTS:
- Vita-Lea: One tablet at breakfast
- Calcium: One tablet at lunch and dinner
- Fiber: One tablespoon Metamucil
- EPA: Three capsules

DAY 3

A woman age 45, who works as a steamstress in a shop that makes seat covers of canvas or other heavy-duty materials. She has two children, 14 and 16. Manual dexterity is essential to her job.

BREAKFAST:
- All-Bran with skim milk and sliced banana. The rest of the family has other cereal and uses low-fat milk.
- Prune juice; other family members have orange juice
- Coffee

LUNCH:
- A "brown bag" lunch, consisting of a sliced turkey breast sandwich using pita bread with Wish-Bone Blue Cheese Dressing and a sliced avocado
- Apple and carrot sticks
- Coffee

MORNING AND AFTERNOON BREAK:
- Bran muffin and coffee

DINNER:
- Burrito with beans, onions, peppers, and sour cream. The children had fried ground beef on their burrito.
- Rice with tomato sauce containing small cubes of green pepper
- Barbequed chicken breast
- Loganberry pie (baked from frozen Mrs. Smith's)

SUPPLEMENTS:
- Vita-Lea: One tablet
- Calcium: Two tablets
- EPA: Six tablets

DAY 4

An executive secretary, 50 years old, with three grown children. She and her husband use her earnings to travel extensively on vacations. The management of her arthritis is important to both of them. The diet prevents the flare-ups that cause discomfort and interfere with her job and lifestyle.

BREAKFAST:
- Omelet made with Egg Beaters, mushrooms, and zucchini sautéed in olive oil with garlic

- Orange juice
- Bran muffin with coffee

LUNCH:
- Salad purchased in cafeteria, consisting of lump salmon in a large, hollowed-out tomato with lots of lemon and shredded lettuce
- Sliced apple
- Hot tea with lemon

MORNING AND AFTERNOON SNACKS:
- Fiber wafers
- Tea (one cup in the morning and one in the afternoon)

DINNER:
- Baked breaded chicken (skin removed before breading)
- Rice boiled and mixed with sautéed vegetables spiced with oregano
- Vegetables (asparagus slices, zucchini, mushroom slices, onion, and garlic clove sautéed in olive oil)
- Small salad of lettuce and cucumber with Italian dressing
- Orange sherbet with sliced oranges

SUPPLEMENTS:
- Vita-Lea: One tablet with breakfast
- Calcium: Three—one with each meal
- EPA: Eight capsules

DAY 5

A "junior executive." He is 36 years of age; his arthritis was diagnosed two years ago. The diet, together with his doctor's support, has helped him reduce his use of medication and his general health has improved.

He is married with three children; everyone in this family plays tennis, likes to swim, and enjoys outdoor activities. His wife follows this diet also.

BREAKFAST:
- Oatmeal with sliced banana and skim milk
- Two bran muffins and coffee

LUNCH:
- Broiled salmon with rice and broccoli at a local restaurant with co-workers. They had wine—he had iced tea.

DINNER:
- Rainbow trout (frozen) sautéed with garlic in olive oil and stuffed with bread chunks and mushrooms (recipe in Chapter 12)
- Long-grain wild rice
- String beans
- Carrot and cabbage salad
- Dessert of lemon chiffon pie
- Chardonnay (one glass)

SUPPLEMENTS:
- Vita-Lea: One tablet at breakfast
- Calcium: Two tablets at dinner
- Vegetable fiber supplement (generic)

DAY 6

A 14-year-old girl who was stricken with arthritis at age 12. Her family has supported her with this dietary commitment. The reinforcement by the family—brothers and sisters—is essential. She is under close medical supervision and on medication.

BREAKFAST:
- Oatmeal with raisins, skim milk, and brown sugar
- One half grapefruit

LUNCH: (Brown bag to school)
- Sandwich: Tuna salad on pita bread with lettuce and avocado (no tomato)
- Apple, sliced for easy eating
- Oatmeal cookies
- Packaged orange drink made from juice

SNACK:
- Popcorn made in microwave—no butter or salt

DINNER:
- Chicken Mango, using skinless chicken breast sliced and sautéed, then cooked briefly with mango and lemon slices
- Brown long-grain rice
- String beans (French cut), broccoli, and pearl onions
- Strawberry chiffon pie with sliced strawberries

SUPPLEMENTS:
- Vita-Lea: One tablet at breakfast
- Calcium: Two tablets at dinner
- EPA: Three capsules before bedtime when they don't cause an aftertaste

DAY 7

Mother of three teenagers and married to an active husband. She has learned to control arthritis completely by diet. This is a Saturday with the entire family.

BREAKFAST:
- Waffles made with Aunt Jemima mix, unprocessed bran, Egg Beaters, and blueberries; maple syrup
- Bran muffin with coffee

LUNCH:
- Barbequed tuna steaks purchased frozen, thawed in a microwave prior to cooking on the charcoal grill
- Salad with chunks of lettuce, celery, zucchini, carrots, green peppers, and cucumbers
- Sliced peaches with yogurt

DINNER:
- Wok-cooked chicken; chicken cut in short strips and cooked quickly in the wok with olive oil and garlic
- Wok-cooked vegetables with pineapple chunks; asparagus, sliced diagonally, alfalfa sprouts, sliced zucchini, grated cabbage, and pineapple chunks cooked quickly in the wok in olive oil. (The chicken is served on top of the vegetables with the pineapple chunks, which are cooked last. The entire dish is served over rice. Use soy sauce if desired.)

SUPPLEMENTS:
- Vita-Lea: Two tablets
- EPA: Two capsules
- Calcium: Three tablets

DAY 8

Sixty-five-year old midwestern homemaker.

Arthritis has been with her since she was about 40 years old. By experimenting with this and other dietary approaches, she has increased her mobility (she bicycles) and has been able to maintain reduced inflammation, and uses medication as necessary. Both she and her husband keep their weight down. She has identified foods to which she is sensitive and they both simply avoid them. She enjoys cooking.

BREAKFAST:
- Oatmeal with yogurt. She mixes the oatmeal with fruit, low-fat yogurt, and wheat germ. She especially likes blueberry yogurt this way. In this way the cereal can be eaten like a classic Bavarian musli, which is a German breakfast food prepared by mixing whole grains with yogurt, nuts, berries, and pieces of dried fruit.
- Bran muffins with prune chunks added before cooking
- Coffee with nondairy creamer

LUNCH:
- Red cabbage, onions, and long sliced carrots all sautéed together in light olive oil
- Lightly sautéed chicken strips served with the cabbage and onions
- Tea

DINNER:
- Frozen fish fillet breaded after thawing by dipping in an egg white and skim milk mix, and then coating with a mixture of flour, dried bread crumbs, and parsley
- Vegetables—lightly steamed broccoli served with boiled white rice
- Apple cake (Chapter 12)
- Tea for her; coffee for him

SUPPLEMENTS:
- Vita-Lea: Two—one tablet in the morning and one in the evening
- Vitamin C: One 500-milligram tablet
- Calcium: Three—one at each meal
- EPA: Four taken at bedtime

DAY 9

A 55-year-old woman who chairs an arthritis support group. Members of this support group meet monthly to help each other cope by sharing things that work, things that don't work; this diet is to some extent an outcome of their participation. She has found from her food diary that she cannot use milk or tomatoes. She has also devised some recipes that many other people have adopted.

BREAKFAST:
- Oatmeal musli: made by mixing cooked oatmeal with apricot nectar, a generous portion of wheat germ, and raisins

LUNCH:
- Pasta salad (Chapter 12)
- Tea or coffee
- Fruit

DINNER:
(All recipes are found in Chapter 12, "Basic Recipes")
- Japanese-style fish steaks
- Red cabbage—high-fiber vegetable dish
- Mushroom rice ring
- Apple cake

SNACKS:
- Popcorn—no butter, moderate salt
- Fiber crackers

SUPPLEMENTS:
- Vita-Lea: One tablet at breakfast and one at dinner
- Calcium: Four tablets
- EPA: Three capsules

DAY 10

A 50-year-old real estate saleswoman. She often puts in 12-hour days and sometimes works seven days a week.

BREAKFAST:
- All-Bran cereal with banana slices and skim milk
- Coffee

MID-MORNING SNACK:
- Coffee

LUNCH:
- Leftover Fish Stew (see Kettle of Fish recipe in Chapter 12)
- Iced tea made from instant mix

DINNER:
- Easy Herb Fish (Chapter 12)
- Leftover braised peas with lettuce (Chapter 12)
- Minute Rice
- Apple cake

SUPPLEMENTS:
- Vita-Lea: One tablet in the morning and one in the evening
- Calcium: Two tablets
- Fiber snacks during the day

DINING OUT

I had a call from one woman on this diet: "Dr. Scala, it's our anniversary and we're going out to dinner; can I go off the diet for one night?" To me that's no problem, but they live in the Midwest and eating out means eating beef. I played dumb. "Why is it necessary to go off the diet?" I queried.

"Well, because I know that my husband will want beef and I'm sure that's what I'll want also."

The conversation slowly changed when I learned that they would be going to a rather expensive restaurant; in fact, the restaurant served live Maine lobsters—expensive, but fine for this diet. I also suggested veal scallopine or veal marsala. But I urged her to try a lobster. I told her it would be an adventure for her, while she gave her husband a night off from her diet, so to speak.

Dining out affords an opportunity to try new things, to give the people around us an opportunity to eat something different. All you have to do is follow the *Do's* and *Don'ts*.

Assert yourself by telling your waiter that you are on a special diet and, if you see something on the menu that looks good, ask questions. For example, in an Italian restaurant ask if they have a pesto sauce, or if their clam sauce is light, without cream. Can sole *meunière* be prepared in olive oil, not butter? The possibilities become endless if you're willing to ask questions and assert your role—that of the customer!

If you live in an area where you're not likely to have a varied menu, call before you go. Ask if they have any nonbeef dishes. Invariably they do; for example, nowadays Midwest restaurants regularly have catfish on their menus; duck is also common, and every restaurant serves chicken in at least one form. If necessary, have a steak, but select a petite filet mignon cooked medium, which will help to remove some of the fat. Add mushrooms sautéed in olive oil (insist!), and a large portion of vegetables—include rice—to increase the carbohydrate content of the diet.

Beyond the entrée, the rest is easy because it's vegetables, rice, fruit, salad, and all things that are on the *Do* list.

Breakfast out is usually the major problem meal. It's only because we Americans seem locked into eggs, bacon, and sausage.

For example, pancakes, waffles, cereal, fruit, toast, even fish are often on the menu. Remember, the amount of egg yolk you get in a serving of pancakes or waffles is not really important. But you must exercise willpower over the meat (such as sausage).

CHAPTER
12 Basic Recipes

Recipes in this chapter will show you how the *Do's* and *Don'ts* work in action.

The recipes range from the easy to prepare to the more complex, which can be served with pride at a gourmet gathering.

You will notice that some of the recipes use butter or margarine. The amount is spread over enough servings that it is not of any consequence. Olive oil or Puritan oil mixed with low-calorie butter substitutes will be even healthier.

The use of some fat and oil in baking is unavoidable. However, try avoiding extensive use of the following:

Animal fats such as bacon fat, butter, lamb fat, lard, and
    poultry fat
Shortenings (except in baking)
Coconut oil
Corn oil and corn oil products
Palm kernel oil
Safflower oil
Soybean oil, hydrogenated
Sunflower oil
Wheat germ oil
Mayonnaise

Butter
Corn oil margarine
Safflower margarine
Soybean margarine
Sandwich spreads such as Miracle Whip
Sandwich spreads from meat and cheese
Peanut butter

Additional recipes can be obtained from cookbooks that emphasize low-fat cooking—fish recipes, vegetarian recipes, and pasta. I urge you to experiment, try new recipes, and exchange recipes with other people who share your commitment.

FIBER RECIPES

Six-Week Bran Muffins

Bran muffins are a great source of fiber. The batter for these muffins will keep for six weeks in the refrigerator. The muffins, if wrapped in plastic and refrigerated, will keep several days up to a week.

1 cup Kellogg's Bran Buds   *1 cup boiling water*

Mix Bran Buds with boiling water and let stand for 10 minutes.

1 cup granulated sugar   *½ teaspoon salt*
½ cup plus 1 tablespoon
  olive oil

Mix together and then stir in:

½ cup Egg Beaters, thawed   *1 pint buttermilk*

Fold in:

2 cups Kellogg's All-Bran   *2½ teaspoons baking soda*
2½ cups flour

Add: Soaked Bran Buds

1 cup raisins

Grease muffin pan.
  Bake muffins at 400° for 15 to 18 minutes.

Yield: 2 quarts batter

Granola Cereal

Granola can be a snack by itself. With milk, it makes an excellent cereal. It is a delicious mix for yogurt, too.

*Soak ¼ cup raisins and 3
   large dates in ½ cup
   water until plump*
*Mash 2 large ripe bananas
   with the soaked raisins
   and dates*
*Stir in 1 tablespoon
   vanilla*

*Mix: 8 cups old-fashioned
   rolled oats*
*½ cup raw, unsalted
   sunflower seeds*
*1 cup chopped walnuts,
   hazelnuts, pine nuts, or
   almonds*
2 teaspoons cinnamon

Add banana mixture to mixed dry ingredients. Spread out on two cookie sheets and bake at 200° until light brown and dry. The mix should be stored dry.

**Yield: about 10 servings as cereal
       unlimited snack**

FISH DISHES

These recipes work best with fresh fish; they are also fine with frozen fish. Unless a specific type of fish is recommended, just use whatever type you prefer.

Easy Herb Fish

Any fish fillets, fresh or frozen can be used. This dish is a snap to prepare and has a wonderful taste.

4 fish fillets (5 or 6 ounces each)
1 clove garlic
1 tablespoon finely chopped onion
½ teaspoon thyme
Pinch oregano
2 tablespoons olive oil
1 tablespoon white wine vinegar

Mix all ingredients except the fish fillets. Spread 1 tablespoon of the mixture on each fillet. Let the fillets stand at room temperature for 30 minutes. Bake the fish at 450° for 8 to 10 minutes in preheated oven. Serve warm with fresh vegetables.

Yield: 4 servings

Seafood Stew

2½ tablespoons butter
1 small onion, chopped
2 stalks celery, including
  tops, chopped
1 large carrot, diced
1 cup water
1 8-ounce can minced
  clams, including juice
1 8-ounce can whole
  baby clams, including
  juice

1 pound fish fillets, cut
  into bite-size pieces
  (ocean perch, haddock,
  sole, etc.)
1 cup nonfat dry milk
1 chicken bouillon cube
2 large potatoes, peeled
  and diced
¼ teaspoon salt
⅛ teaspoon black pepper
Dash celery salt

Melt butter in large saucepan. Sauté onion, celery, and carrot until onion is tender. Stir in water, clams, fish, milk powder, and bouillon cube. Add potatoes and seasonings; cover. Simmer over very low heat about 20 minutes or until potatoes are tender. Do not allow to boil.

Yield: 4 to 6 servings

Sole Véronique

1 cup seedless green grapes,
halved
2 tablespoons dry white wine
1 pound sole fillets
1 tablespoon lemon juice
Salt and black pepper to
taste

½ teaspoon grated orange
peel
1 teaspoon diet margarine
1 orange, cut in slices
Watercress sprigs

Place grapes in bowl and drizzle with wine. Arrange fish on a sheet of aluminum foil on a broiling pan, and sprinkle with lemon juice. Season with salt, pepper, and grated orange peel. Dot with diet margarine. Broil until golden brown, about 5 minutes. Arrange the wine-marinated grapes, cut side down, over the top of the sole fillets, and broil about 1 minute longer. Garnish each serving with an orange slice and watercress.

Yield: 4 servings

Red Snapper

½ cup chopped onions
Olive oil
1 #2½ can whole
tomatoes
Salt and black pepper to
taste
2 pounds red snapper
fillets

1 2-ounce jar pimiento,
coarsely chopped
2 tablespoons capers
1 3-ounce jar green olives,
drained and sliced

Cook onions in olive oil until wilted. Add tomatoes, salt, and pepper; cook 5 minutes.

Place red snapper in buttered casserole dish.

Sprinkle pimiento, capers, and green olives on top; pour sauce over this.

Bake at 350° for 25 to 30 minutes.

Yield: 6 servings

Japanese-Style Grilled Fish Steaks

*4 1-inch thick fish
steaks (halibut, salmon,
swordfish)*
*¼ cup low-sodium lite soy
sauce*
*3 tablespoons minced
onion*

*1 tablespoon peeled and
chopped fresh ginger*
*1 tablespoon toasted
sesame seeds*
*½ teaspoon granulated
sugar*

Rinse the fish steaks and pat dry; place them in a single layer in a shallow pan. Put soy sauce, onion, ginger, sesame seeds, and sugar into a blender container; blend on low speed for 30 seconds, scraping the sides down once. Pour the sauce over the fish and turn to coat both sides. Marinate for 30 minutes, turning the fish occasionally. Remove fish from marinade and place on an oiled grill 4 inches from moderately hot coals. Cook for 5 minutes on each side, or until the fish flakes when tested with a fork.

If using a broiler, place the fish 4 inches from the broiler (or flame); cook 4 minutes and turn. Then cook 3 minutes on second side or until tender.

Yield: 4 servings

Yogurt-Sauced Fish

Yogurt Sauce

1 cup plain yogurt
2 tablespoons all-purpose
  flour

2 teaspoons grated lemon rind
1 small onion, minced
¾ teaspoon salt

Mix yogurt, flour, lemon rind, onion, and salt in small bowl.

Fish

1½ pounds mild whitefish
  (whitefish, ocean perch,
  haddock, etc.)

¼ teaspoon paprika
Dash freshly ground black
  pepper

Place fish in a shallow 2-quart baking dish; pour yogurt sauce on top. Sprinkle paprika and pepper over sauce.

Bake at 350° for 20 to 30 minutes or just until tender. Do not overcook.

Yield: 4 to 6 servings

Kettle of Fish

3 large potatoes, peeled and
   thinly sliced
Salt
½ pound fresh mushrooms,
   sliced
1 pound zucchini, in
   ⅛-inch slices
4 large tomatoes, peeled,
   seeded, and sliced
2 green onions, thinly
   sliced

1½ pounds fish fillets
   (haddock, sole, or
   flounder)
2 tablespoons butter,
   melted
½ teaspoon thyme
½ teaspoon basil
½ teaspoon oregano
Black pepper to taste
Parsley and lemon slices

Generously grease a 2-quart oblong baking dish. Arrange
potatoes on the bottom and sprinkle with salt. Cover with foil
and bake at 350° for 15 minutes. Place vegetables over
partially cooked potatoes; then arrange fish fillets over vegetables. Cut a few diagonal slashes in fish. Dribble melted
butter over fish and sprinkle with herbs, more salt, and dash
black pepper. Bake 20 minutes more or until fish is browned
slightly and flakes. Garnish with parsley and lemon slices.

Yield: 4 to 6 servings

Baked Trout with Mushrooms

Even though this recipe was created for a whole blue-skinned fish such as trout (about 10 to 12 inches), it can also be used with freshwater coho salmon or ocean salmon of similar size. Alternatively, try a segment of a large, whole salmon.

*4 trout, cleaned with heads
  and tails left on*
*Salt and freshly ground
  black pepper*
Flour
½ cup butter
2 tablespoons olive oil

*1 pound fresh mushrooms,
  thinly sliced*
1 teaspoon lemon juice
*¾ cup thinly sliced green
  onions (include 2 or 3
  inches of green stem)*
¼ cup fresh bread crumbs

Season trout lightly with salt and pepper. Roll in flour and brush off excess. In a heavy 10- to 12-inch skillet, melt 2 tablespoons of the butter with the olive oil over high heat. When foam subsides, add the trout and cook for 4 to 5 minutes on each side until golden brown. Carefully transfer trout to a platter. In a stainless steel or enamel skillet, melt 4 tablespoons of the butter over moderate heat. Add mushrooms and sprinkle with lemon juice. Cook until soft, about 3 minutes, while turning with a wooden spoon. Remove mushrooms to a buttered 9 × 13 inch baking dish. Put 1 tablespoon of the butter in skillet and add green onions. Cook 1 minute. Remove to a bowl. Lightly brown bread crumbs in remaining butter. Place trout on mushrooms, then top with green onions and bread crumbs. Bake at 425° for about 10 minutes, or until trout is white and flakes.

Yield: 4 servings

Tuna Salad

1 12½-ounce can tuna, drained
1 cup chopped celery
1 cup alfalfa sprouts
½ cup Egg Beater mayonnaise
1 cup shredded carrots

⅔ cup thinly sliced green onion
⅓ cup peeled and chopped cucumber
2 teaspoons lemon juice
3 tablespoons pickle relish

Place tuna in a medium bowl and flake it. Mix in remaining ingredients. This tuna salad may be refrigerated overnight. For a light and pretty meal, fill a tomato with this nutritious salad.

Yield: 4 cups

White Clam Sauce

3 tablespoons olive oil
1 small onion, minced
2 cloves garlic, minced
2 8-ounce cans minced clams

½ cup dry white wine
1 tablespoon minced fresh parsley
¼ teaspoon white pepper
2 tablespoons butter

Heat oil in skillet. Add onion and garlic. Sauté in oil over medium heat until golden. Drain clam liquid into onion mixture. Stir in wine. Simmer about 5 minutes over medium heat. Stir in clams, parsley, pepper, and butter; heat thoroughly. Pour clam sauce over hot cooked vermicelli, linguine, or spaghetti.

Yield: 4 or 5 servings

POULTRY AND GAME DISHES

Some people have difficulty shifting from a diet rich in red meat to a diet that emphasizes fish and fowl. These recipes will help to make the transition enjoyable.

Chicken with Broccoli and Cashews

1 tablespoon cornstarch
1 cup chicken broth
3 tablespoons dry sherry
2 tablespoons soy sauce
¼ to ½ teaspoon Tabasco
  sauce
¼ cup olive oil
3 chicken breasts, skinned,
  boned, and cut into
  1-inch chunks
2 slices peeled fresh ginger
  (½ teaspoon powdered)

3 cups broccoli flowerets
1 medium sweet red
  pepper, cut in 1-inch
  squares
½ pound mushrooms,
  sliced
1 bunch green onions,
  slivered
1 clove garlic, minced
⅓ cup dry-roasted cashews

Combine the cornstarch, chicken broth, sherry, soy sauce, and Tabasco in a small bowl and have ready.

Ten minutes before serving, heat olive oil in a hot skillet or wok. When oil is very hot, add chicken and ginger. Cook about 3 minutes, stirring constantly, until chicken turns white. If using a skillet, remove chicken and discard ginger slices. If using a wok, remove ginger slices and push chicken up sides.

Place broccoli, red pepper, mushrooms, green onions, and minced garlic in the skillet or center of wok. Cook 3 minutes, stirring constantly.

Combine the chicken and the cornstarch mixture with the vegetables and continue stirring until the sauce thickens slightly. Sprinkle in the cashews and serve immediately with steaming hot rice.

Yield: 6 servings

Lemon Chicken Brochettes

1½ pounds boned and
  skinned chicken breasts

3 small zucchini, unpeeled
½ pound whole mushrooms

Cut breasts across the grain into 2-inch wide pieces. Slice zucchini 1 inch thick. Alternate chicken, zucchini, and mushrooms on 4 skewers, keeping everything about the same thickness for even cooking, and place these in a shallow glass dish for marinating.

Marinade

Juice of 3 lemons
1 tablespoon grated lemon
  peel
¼ cup olive oil
1 tablespoon granulated
  sugar

1 tablespoon cider vinegar
1 clove garlic, minced
2 teaspoons salt
¼ teaspoon cayenne pepper

Combine the preceding ingredients, and pour over brochettes. Cover and let sit at room temperature for 1 to 2 hours, turning periodically. (Refrigerate if they are to sit any longer.)

Slowly barbecue brochettes over medium coals for 25 to 30 minutes, turning periodically. Baste with marinade. Serve on beds of rice, holding meat down with a fork while withdrawing skewers. Provide individual bowls of the following butter sauce for dipping.

Butter Sauce

¼ cup melted butter
1 tablespoon lemon juice

1 tablespoon chopped parsley
Dash cayenne pepper

Yield: 4 servings

Chicken Tahitian

2 teaspoons salt
1 teaspoon paprika
1 teaspoon curry powder
8 to 10 split chicken
  breasts
4 tablespoons flour

6 tablespoons butter
1½ cups pineapple chunks;
  reserve juice
1½ cups canned seedless
  grapes

Mix salt, paprika, curry powder, and flour; sprinkle over chicken. Add butter to pan and brown chicken. Set aside.

Sauce

1 cup orange juice
½ cup white wine vinegar
1 cup lemon juice
⅔ cup brown sugar
1 cup water

1 cup white wine
1 cup pineapple juice
2 teaspoons curry powder
7 tablespoons flour
Salt and black pepper

Combine all sauce ingredients and simmer 10 minutes, stirring with whisk or until sauce thickens. Pour over chicken in baking dish; bake covered, at 350°, for 45 minutes. Add pineapple and grapes during the last 10 minutes.

Yield: 8 to 10 servings

Chicken with Basil

*3 to 4 tablespoons seeded
and finely chopped
canned California green
chilies*
2 tablespoons soy sauce
*1 teaspoon each sugar and
vinegar*
*½ cup coarsely chopped
fresh basil or 2
tablespoons dried basil*
*1 teaspoon chopped fresh
or dried mint*

½ teaspoon cornstarch
3 tablespoons olive oil
*2 whole chicken breasts
(about 1 pound each),
skinned, boned, and cut in
strips ¼ inch thick and 2
inches long*
*1 clove garlic, minced or
mashed*
*1 large onion, halved,
then sliced ¼ inch thick*

Mix together chilies, soy sauce, sugar, vinegar, basil, mint, and cornstarch; set aside.

Heat 2 tablespoons of the olive oil in a large skillet or wok over high heat. When oil is hot, add the chicken and garlic; cook, stirring constantly, until meat loses pinkness (about 4 minutes); then turn out of pan. Heat another 1 tablespoon oil, then add onion; cook, stirring, for 1 minute. Add chili mixture and return chicken and its juices to pan; cook, stirring, until sauce thickens slightly.

Yield: 3 or 4 servings

Citrus Chicken Breasts

4 whole chicken breasts,
halved, skinned, and
boned
½ teaspoon salt

½ teaspoon paprika
½ teaspoon dried basil
¼ teaspoon dried rosemary
¼ teaspoon black pepper

Mix together and sprinkle over the chicken.

1 tablespoon butter
3 tablespoons fresh lemon
juice
3 tablespoons lime juice

3 tablespoons orange juice
¼ cup white wine
3 tablespoons low-fat
yogurt

Melt butter in skillet; add seasoned chicken and brown on both sides (about 5 minutes).

Mix citrus juices and wine. Pour over chicken in pan. Cover and simmer about 15 minutes, or until tender.

Remove chicken to warm dish. Into the liquid in pan slowly stir in the yogurt. Heat about 1 minute; then pour over chicken.

Yield: 8 servings

Chicken Salad with Rice and Almonds

3 to 3½ pounds chicken
  breasts, cooked, skinned,
  boned, and diced
1 cup diced celery
1 bunch green onions,
  finely chopped (white
  part only)
1 cup diced jicama
  (optional)
8 cherry tomatoes,
  quartered

1 cup coarsely chopped
  almonds
⅓ cup minced parsley
3 cups cooked brown rice
½ cup olive oil
Juice of 1 large lemon
2 teaspoons dried oregano
Salt and freshly ground
  black pepper

Combine chicken, celery, green onions, jicama, tomatoes, almonds, and parsley. Toss together to mix well; then stir in rice a little at a time to mix well.

Combine oil, lemon juice, and oregano in a small jar with a tight-fitting lid; shake well, pour over salad and toss. Add more lemon juice if desired. Season with salt and black pepper to taste.

Yield: 5 to 6 servings

Roast Duck

4- to 5-pound duckling
Salt
Lemon pepper
4 oranges
1 lemon
4 onions, quartered
1 bay leaf
Pinch dried thyme and
  rosemary

2 stalks celery, chopped
2 carrots, chopped
½ cup granulated sugar
2 teaspoons white cider
  vinegar
2 teaspoons tomato puree
2 cups chicken broth
1 jigger brandy

Remove pin feathers of duck and singe the duck if necessary. Rinse duck and giblets with cold water. Drain. Rub with salt and lemon pepper.

Stuff into the cavity of the duck slices of rind from the oranges and lemon and one quartered onion. Place duck breast side up in roasting pan, surrounded with giblets, bay leaf, thyme, rosemary, celery, carrots, and remaining onions.

Roast duck in a 450° oven. After 1 hour reduce heat to 350°. Continue roasting, until duck is brown and tender (about 1 hour), then transfer to another pan or plate and split the whole length of the back. Remove all the bones except drumsticks. Keep warm. Save 2 or 3 slices of orange rind for garnish.

Squeeze juice from the oranges and lemon.

In a saucepan heat the sugar with the vinegar to carmelize; add citrus juices, tomato puree, and chicken broth. Skim all fat from roasting pan and pour in the sauce. Simmer to reduce; add the brandy. Cover duck with sauce and garnish with a few orange rind slices.

Yield: 4 servings

Glazed Duck with Peanut-Rice Stuffing

1 cup chopped celery
1/2 cup chopped onions
1 teaspoon each salt and
    black pepper
1/2 cup olive oil
2 1/2 cups cooked white rice
2 cups chopped peanuts
    (dry roasted)

1/4 cup chopped parsley
1/2 teaspoon dried rosemary
1 cup orange juice
1 cup orange sections
Grated orange peel
2 4- to 5-pound ducklings
1/4 cup honey
2 teaspoons soy sauce

Sauté celery, onions, salt, and pepper in olive oil slowly until tender. Then toss together with rice and peanuts. Add parsley, rosemary, orange juice, orange sections, and orange peel to the preceding mixture.

Stuff each duckling with half of mixture. Skewer opening and truss.

Roast on rack in 350° oven 25 to 30 minutes per pound.

Combine honey and soy sauce. Brush evenly over surface of duckling 30 minutes before removing from oven.

Yield: 4 to 6 servings

Rabbit in Red Wine

1 large frying rabbit, cut in
   serving-size pieces
½ cup flour
1 teaspoon salt
½ teaspoon coarsely
   ground black pepper
2 tablespoons olive oil
1 tablespoon butter
6 to 8 small boiling
   onions, peeled

4 to 6 garlic cloves,
   minced
1 bay leaf
¼ teaspoon each thyme
   and rosemary
6 to 8 mushrooms,
   quartered
1 cup dry red wine
1 cup chicken broth

Dust rabbit pieces with a mixture of flour, salt, and pepper. Heat olive oil and butter in a heavy skillet; brown rabbit pieces in it, a few at a time, turning often to brown them evenly on all sides. Then set them aside. Brown the onions and garlic lightly in the same pan, adding a bit more butter if needed. Add bay leaf, thyme, rosemary, and mushrooms; toss and cook for a minute or two. Pour in the wine and chicken broth; then bring to a boil while scraping the pan to incorporate any browned bits clinging to the bottom and sides.

Place the rabbit pieces back in the pan, cover, and simmer over low heat for 30 minutes. Remove rabbit to a warm platter and pour sauce on top.

Yield: 4 to 6 servings

Salmon Omelet

1 7½-ounce can salmon
2 tablespoons chopped
  parsley
1 teaspoon minced onion

Lemon pepper
1 cup Egg Beaters
Pinch cream of tartar
2 teaspoons margarine

Mix salmon, parsley, onion, and lemon pepper.

Combined Egg Beaters and cream of tartar in the small bowl of an electric mixer. Beat for 5 minutes at high speed. Fold in salmon mixture.

Melt margarine over medium-high heat in heavy skillet or omelet pan with ovenproof handle. Pour in preceding mixture. Heat without stirring just until bottom is set. Place skillet in preheated 325° oven for about 5 minutes or until completely set. Then loosen edges of omelet with spatula. Fold in half. Lift out onto serving plate. Serve with dill sauce.

Yield: 2 servings

Dill Sauce

Melt 1 tablespoon margarine in saucepan. Stir in 1 tablespoon flour, 1 teaspoon dill (fresh if possible), and dash lemon pepper. Gradually add ⅔ cup skim milk. Bring to boil, stirring constantly. Boil 1 minute.

EGG DISHES

Egg Beaters provide the means for egg lovers to enjoy their favorite food while following my plan. I have included two recipes, which are both tasty and illustrative of what can be done with Egg Beaters to make an interesting meal.

Spinach-Onion Quiche

1 cup flour (unsifted)
1 teaspoon salt
½ cup margarine

2 to 3 tablespoons cold
water

Combine flour and salt; add margarine and beat with electric beater. Add water, mix with cold fork, and form into a ball. Avoid handling and use only necessary amount of water.

Roll out dough to fit a 9-inch pie pan; flute edges. Spread foil in pan, cover with dried beans to weight down.

Bake in 400° oven for 10 minutes. Remove foil and beans. Set pastry aside.

Filling

¾ cup chopped onion
2 tablespoons margarine
1 10-ounce package frozen
  leaf spinach
Sauté onion but do not
  brown. Thaw spinach
  (dip in boiling water),
  drain, and cut up. Add
  onion to spinach and
  spread on pastry shell.

1 cup Egg Beaters
1 cup skim milk
¼ teaspoon black pepper
  and salt
Pinch nutmeg

Combine all ingredients and mix into spinach mixture.

Bake at 375° for 30 minutes or until knife inserted in center comes out clean. Let stand 10 minutes before serving.

Yield: 8 generous servings

VEGETABLE DISHES

There are, of course, numerous ways to cook vegetables. The recipes emphasize methods that impart special taste and variety. I cannot emphasize enough the variety of vegetables available and that variety is important to good health.

Red Cabbage

1 to 1½ pounds red cabbage (remove outer leaves), sliced in wedges
½ large onion, chopped
2 tablespoons olive oil
Pinch lemon pepper

⅛ to ¼ cup white cider vinegar
2 tablespoons brown sugar
1 large or 2 medium apples (cored and sliced, with skins on)

Sauté onion in olive oil in a 10-inch skillet with cover or until softened, 3 to 5 minutes; stir; add lemon pepper; then stir in vinegar, sugar, and apple; cover with cabbage. Cook slowly, covered, for 10 to 15 minutes, stirring occasionally.

Yield: 4 to 6 servings

Gingered Carrots

7 to 8 medium carrots
1 tablespoon sugar
1 teaspoon cornstarch
¼ teaspoon salt

¼ teaspoon powdered ginger
¼ cup orange juice
2 tablespoons olive oil
Chopped parsley

Cut carrots on the bias into ⅛- to ¼-inch thick slices. Cook, covered, in boiling salted water until just tender, about 7 to 10 minutes. Drain.

Combine sugar, cornstarch, salt, and ginger in a small saucepan. Add orange juice and cook, stirring constantly, until mixture thickens and bubbles. Boil 1 minute, then stir in olive oil. Pour over hot carrots and toss. Garnish with chopped parsley.

Yield: 6 servings

Braised Peas with Lettuce

2 cups shredded lettuce
2 cups shelled green peas
  (2 pounds unshelled) or
  two 10-ounce packages
  frozen petite peas
¼ cup sliced green onions
1 teaspoon sugar

¼ teaspoon salt
¼ teaspoon dried summer
  savory or ¾ teaspoon
  fresh
⅛ teaspoon white pepper
2 tablespoons olive oil

Place 1 cup of the shredded lettuce in a large saucepan. Top with the peas and green onions. Sprinkle with sugar, salt, savory, and white pepper. Sprinkle with olive oil and top with the remaining 1 cup lettuce. Cover tightly and cook over medium-low heat for 5 to 10 minutes, until the peas are tender.

Yield: 4 servings

Carrots in Mint Sauce

*6 carrots, diced, sliced, or
    slivered*
⅓ cup reserved liquid
2 tablespoons butter
*1 tablespoon granulated
    sugar*

1 teaspoon cornstarch
⅛ teaspoon salt
*Juice and grated rind of ½
    lemon*
*1 tablespoon finely chopped
    mint leaves*

Parboil carrots, covered, in a small amount of boiling, salted water for 4 to 8 minutes; reserve ⅓ cup of the liquid. Melt butter in a medium saucepan. Combine sugar, cornstarch, and salt and stir into melted butter. Add lemon, mint, and reserved liquid. Stir until just thickened. When ready to serve, add carrots to heated sauce and toss to glaze.

Yield: 4 servings

Stuffed Acorn Squash

*2 acorn squash, halved and
    seeded*
3 tablespoons olive oil
1 cup grated carrot

*½ cup chopped pitted
    prunes*
¼ cup chopped dates
¼ teaspoon nutmeg

Place squash cut side down in baking pan with small amount of water. Bake at 350° for 30 minutes.

Combine remaining ingredients. Turn squash cut side up and fill with prune-date mixture. Bake 25 to 30 minutes more, or until squash is tender.

Yield: 4 servings

Mushroom–Rice Ring

1 cup chopped mushrooms
2 tablespoons olive oil
¼ teaspoon nutmeg

5 to 6 cups cooked
long-grain white rice

In a medium skillet, sauté the chopped mushrooms in the olive oil until tender but not brown. Season with nutmeg.

Combined mushrooms and rice and turn into a well-buttered, 5- to 6-cup ring mold, pressing mixture down gently. Turn out at once on a warm serving plate to keep the mold warm in a pan of hot water until ready to serve.

Surround the rice ring and fill its center with green vegetables such as Chinese pea pods or broccoli.

Yield: 6 to 8 servings

Ratatouille

1 medium eggplant
1 tablespoon salt
¼ cup olive oil
2 large onions, sliced
3 cloves garlic, crushed
1 medium red pepper
  (optional), cored and
  cubed
1 medium green pepper,
  cored and cubed
4 medium zucchini, sliced
  ¾ inch thick

3 medium tomatoes, peeled,
  seeded, and cubed
¼ teaspoon salt
Freshly ground black
  pepper to taste
¼ teaspoon dried thyme
¼ teaspoon dried oregano
1 bay leaf
2 tablespoons chopped
  fresh parsley

Cut eggplant into ½-inch thick slices, then into cubes. Sprinkle with 1 tablespoon salt and let stand 30 minutes; then pat dry with paper towels.

Heat olive oil in large skillet. Sauté onions and garlic 2 minutes. Add peppers; cook 2 minutes. Add eggplant cubes and brown lightly, about 3 minutes; turn them often. Add zucchini, tomatoes, and all the seasonings but parsley. Simmer gently, uncovered, 30 to 40 minutes, until all vegetables are just tender. Baste vegetables often; do not let them scorch. Cover; reduce heat if necessary. Remove bay leaf, put ratatouille in a serving bowl, and garnish with parsley. May be served hot or cold.

Yield: 8 to 10 servings

Green Beans with Mushroom Sauce

3 cups French-style green
beans

Mushroom Sauce

2 cups sliced mushrooms
3 tablespoons butter
2 teaspoons all-purpose
flour

¼ teaspooon salt
Black pepper to taste
½ cup plain yogurt

Cook beans in boiling water until tender.

Sauté mushrooms in butter in a deep skillet until just soft. Stir in flour, salt, and pepper; cook and stir until flour absorbs mushroom juices and thickens. Remove from heat and stir in yogurt. Add beans; warm slightly, but do not boil.

Yield: 4 servings

Wheat and Ginger Broccoli

¼ cup butter
1 clove garlic, minced
½ teaspoon salt
½ teaspoon powdered
ginger

2 tablespoons wheat germ
3 cups fresh broccoli, cut
into bite-size pieces,
cooked until tender-crisp

Melt butter in skillet; sauté garlic until tender. Add salt, ginger, and wheat germ. Stir-fry quickly until well mixed and wheat germ is just browned, being careful not to burn mixture. Add broccoli; stir to coat. Heat through.

Yield: 4 to 6 servings

Stir-fried Green Beans

2 tablespoons olive oil
½ pound fresh green
  beans, cut diagonally
  into 1½-inch lengths
1 clove garlic, minced

½ cup chicken broth
¼ teaspoon granulated
  sugar
Salt and black pepper

Heat a wok; add oil and swish to coat sides; heat briefly.

Add beans with garlic. Stir-fry 30 seconds to coat beans with oil. Add broth, bring to boil, reduce to low heat. Cover and cook 8 minutes, stirring occasionally. Beans should be bright green and crunchy.

Remove cover, add sugar and a pinch of salt and black pepper. Stir to blend.

Yield: 2 or 3 servings

Stir-fried Vegetables

2 tablespoons olive oil
1 cup thinly sliced carrots
1 cup quartered mushrooms
½ cup sliced water
  chestnuts
2 large cloves garlic,
  minced
2 cups fresh Chinese pea
  pods or 1 package frozen,
  partly thawed pea pods

1 large cucumber, sliced in
  half lengthwise, seeds
  removed and cut into
  strips about 3 inches by
  ¼ inch
1 can chicken broth
2 tablespoons dry sherry or
  white wine
1 tablespoon soy sauce

Heat a wok or skillet for 2 minutes. Add olive oil and heat briefly. Quickly add carrots, mushrooms, water chestnuts, and garlic. Stir-fry 6 minutes. Push foods to one side of wok. Add pea pods and cucumbers. Cook 3 minutes, stirring constantly.

Push pea pods to side, add broth, wine, and soy sauce. Then return all vegetables and cook another 3 minutes. Remove vegetables with strainer and serve.

Substitute whole fresh or frozen green beans if pea pods are unavailable.

Apples and Yams

3 cups thinly sliced apples,
  unpeeled
1 to 2 pounds fresh yams,
  cooked and sliced

½ cup packed brown sugar
¼ teaspoon cinnamon
3 tablespoons melted
  butter

Remove skin from yams; arrange apples and yams in shallow casserole.

Combine brown sugar, cinnamon, and melted butter and pour over casserole.

Bake at 350° about 30 minutes, basting occasionally.

Gardener's Salad

*½ pound spaghetti, broken
  into thirds and cooked,
  or ½ pound cooked noodles*
*1½ cups cooked chicken,
  cut into strips*
*1 cup red cabbage, finely
  shredded*
*½ cup cauliflowerets,
  parboiled and sliced*

½ cup ripe olives, sliced
*3 tablespoons chopped red
  onion*
*1 2-ounce jar diced
  pimiento*
½ cup Italian dressing
*2 tablespoons chopped
  parsley*

Combine all ingredients with cooked spaghetti or noodles.
Mix well and chill.

Toss again before serving on bed of lettuce.

SALADS

Salads enhance eating pleasure. Some of these make wonderful vegetarian meals by themselves, and others add appeal
to a meal that emphasizes fish or fowl.

Carrot and Cabbage Salad

1 package lemon Jell-O
1 cup boiling water
½ cup cold water
½ cup lemon juice

*¼ head green cabbage,
  shredded*
4 carrots, shredded

Dissolve Jell-O in boiling water; then add cold water and
lemon juice. Refrigerate until slightly jelled.

Stir in shredded cabbage and carrots and refrigerate until
firmly set.

Pasta Salad

4 cups cooked bite-size pasta
   of any kind such as
   shells, bows, or twists
2 tablespoons olive oil
½ cup pesto dressing (see
   below)

1 head leaf lettuce
1 red pepper, seeded and
   cut into rings
½ cup thin cucumber slices
3 tablespoons pine nuts

Toss cooked pasta with olive oil. Add pesto dressing and toss until pasta is well coated. Arrange pasta on a bed of lettuce and garnish with pepper rings and cucumber slices. Top each serving with pine nuts.

Yield: 4 servings

Pesto Dressing

2 tablespoons white wine
   vinegar
1 tablespoon Dijon mustard
1 clove garlic, finely
   chopped
Salt and black pepper

1 tablespoon water
¾ cup olive oil
3 tablespoons finely
   chopped fresh basil
2 tablespoons grated
   Parmesan cheese

Put vinegar, mustard, garlic, salt, pepper, and water into a small bowl. Beat well with a fork or whisk. Beat in oil, a little at a time. When thick and emulsified, stir in basil and cheese. Let stand for 30 minutes before using, to enhance the flavor.

Yield: One cup

Spinach Salad

Salad Dressing

2 tablespoons olive oil
Juice of 1 lemon
1 tablespoon Dijon mustard
1 tablespoon grated
  Parmesan cheese

1 teaspoon sugar
1 teaspoon Worcestershire
  sauce
½ teaspoon salt
Dash black pepper

Combine all ingredients in small jar with lid. Shake well; chill.

Salad

10 ounces fresh spinach
¼ pound fresh mushrooms,
  sliced

1 hard-cooked egg white,
  sieved or chopped
¼ cup sunflower seeds

Thoroughly wash spinach, tear into bite-size pieces, and chill in tight plastic bag to crisp. Combine spinach and mushrooms in large bowl and toss with dressing. Garnish with egg white and sunflower seeds.

Yield: 4 servings

Apple Cabbage Salad

Yogurt Salad Dressing

1 tablespoon cider vinegar
1 teaspoon caraway seeds
1 teaspoon prepared
  mustard

½ teaspoon salt
⅛ teaspoon garlic salt
1 cup plain yogurt

Combine vinegar and spices. Fold into yogurt; cover. Chill several hours.

Salad

2 medium red apples,
  unpeeled, chopped coarsely
1 teaspoon lemon juice
2 cups shredded green cabbage

2 cups shredded red
  cabbage
¾ cup finely chopped celery

Sprinkle apples with lemon juice. When ready to serve, mix yogurt dressing with apples, cabbages, and celery.

Yield: 6 to 8 servings

Chef's Salad

½ head Boston lettuce
1 large tomato, cut into
　eighths
½ cucumber, thinly sliced

1 small onion, grated
½ green pepper, cut into
　thin strips

Wash lettuce; tear into bite-size pieces. Arrange on salad platter with tomato, cucumber, onion, and green pepper. Cover; refrigerate while preparing dressing and remaining ingredients.

Salad Dressing

½ cup plain yogurt
1 tablespoon lemon juice
½ teaspoon salt
⅛ teaspoon white pepper

1 clove garlic, minced
1 teaspoon chopped parsley
1 teaspoon dried dill

Blend yogurt with lemon juice; season with salt, pepper, garlic, parsley, and dill. Pour dressing over greens.
　For the top of the salad:

1 cup cooked chicken, cut
　into julienne strips
2 sardines, drained, cut in
　half lengthwise

3 stuffed green olives,
　sliced

Arrange chicken and sardines on top of salad. Garnish with sliced olives.

Yield: 4 servings

Mandarin Orange Salad

*2 heads red lettuce (or 3
  heads butter lettuce)*
½ cup chopped celery
⅓ cup sliced green onions
½ cup watercress sprigs

¼ cup chopped parsley
*1 11-ounce can mandarin
  oranges, drained*
*½ cup chopped walnuts,
  almonds, or pecans*

Dress with the following just before serving:

½ cup olive oil
¼ cup tarragon vinegar
*2 tablespoons granulated
  sugar*
*½ teaspoon Worcestershire
  sauce*

1 teaspoon salt
*Freshly ground black
  pepper to taste*
*Dash Tabasco sauce
  (optional)*

With a whisk, beat the preceding ingredients together thoroughly until sugar is dissolved.

Note: Delicious substitutions are grapefruit and avocado slices in place of the mandarin oranges, and pine nuts instead of walnuts.

Golden Coleslaw

2 cups apple cider vinegar
2 cups sugar
*2 to 3 heads cabbage,
  shredded*
1 teaspoon turmeric
1½ teaspoons mustard seed

1½ teaspoons celery seed
Chopped onion
Chopped green pepper
Pimiento to color
Salt to flavor

Boil vinegar and sugar 1 minute. Combine all ingredients and mix well. This coleslaw will keep 3 weeks in tightly closed container in the refrigerator.

Fresh Vegetable Salad Platter

*2 9-ounce packages frozen
    whole green beans*
*1 large cucumber, pared
    and thinly sliced*
*1 medium green pepper,
    cut into 1-inch long
    julienne strips*

1 cup sliced radishes
½ cup sliced green onions
*1 head Boston lettuce,
    washed and crisped*

Dressing

¾ cup olive oil
*6 tablespoons tarragon
    vinegar*
*3 tablespoons lime or
    lemon juice*

4 teaspoons sugar
1½ teaspoons salt
¼ teaspoon black pepper

Combine ingredients for dressing in jar with tight-fitting lid. Shake vigorously to blend.

Cook green beans as package label directs; drain. In medium bowl, toss with half the dressing, then refrigerate, covered, tossing occasionally until well chilled, at least 2 hours. Also chill cucumber, green pepper, radishes, green onions, and remaining dressing.

To serve, line shallow bowl with lettuce leaves. Mound green beans in center; arrange vegetables decoratively around edge. Shake chilled dressing well, then pour over salad and toss.

Yield: 10 servings

Navel Orange and Kiwi Salad

Serve in orange halves or as slices on individual plates.

*2 medium-size carrots,
  shredded*
¼ cup orange juice
*3 kiwis, peeled (make 12
  pieces out of 3)*

*3 large navel oranges, cut
  in half*
Parsley to garnish
*½ cup plain low-fat yogurt
  (optional)*

Combine shredded carrots with orange juice.

If oranges are used as shells, cut around segments but leave in place. Overlap 2 kiwi slices on top of each orange half.

Spoon one-sixth of carrot mixture onto top of each orange.

If oranges are sliced on individual plates, alternate orange slices and kiwi slices and carrot mixture as above on individual plates. Offer yogurt if you want an additional contrast.

Yield: 6 servings

Apple Yogurt Salad

1 cup low-fat plain yogurt
*1½ tablespoons lemon
  juice*
½ teaspoon cinnamon
*1 to 2 tablespoons honey
  or brown sugar*

*3 large red Delicious
  apples, unpeeled and
  thinly sliced*
*4 tablespoons chopped
  walnuts*
4 tablespoons chopped dates

Stir first four ingredients together well and add thinly sliced apples. Mix gently to coat evenly.

Line 6 or 8 salad plates with crisp lettuce. Arrange coated apple slices on top. Spoon any leftover dressing over apples.

Sprinkle chopped dates and nuts over the top.

Yield: 6 to 8 servings

DRESSINGS

These dressings and mayonnaises permit you to follow my diet without sacrificing flavor or texture. They are also helpful in adapting traditional foods to this commitment. For example, with Egg Beater mayonnaise you can have a tuna sandwich with all the benefit of tuna and without the detriment of egg yolks.

Egg Beater Mayonnaise

1/3 cup Egg Beaters
1/2 teaspoon dry mustard
1/2 teaspoon granulated
   sugar

1/4 teaspoon paprika
2 tablespoons white
   vinegar
1 cup olive oil

Combine Egg Beaters, mustard, sugar, paprika, vinegar, and 1/2 cup of the olive oil in blender container. Blend on medium-high speed until mixed. Without turning off blender, pour in remaining oil in a slow, steady stream. If necessary, use rubber spatula to keep mixture flowing to blades. Continue blending until oil is completely incorporated and mixture is smooth and thick.

Yield: 1½ cups

Soybean Mayonnaise

6 ounces tofu (soybean
   curd); press between
   towels to remove liquid

5 teaspoons lemon or lime
   juice
3 tablespoons olive oil

Blend tofu and juice together and add oil slowly. Then blend on medium-low speed in blender.
   Store tightly; it is best after 4 days.

Yield: 1 cup

Orange Salad Dressing

¼ cup orange juice
1 to 2 teaspoons grated
 orange peel
2 tablespoons cider vinegar

1 envelope Italian salad
 dressing mix
⅔ cup olive oil

Put orange juice, orange peel, cider vinegar, and salad dressing mix in a bottle; cover and shake well. Pour in olive oil, cover, and shake well. Chill.
 Shake dressing before using.

Yield: 1 cup salad dressing

This recipe is good with carrot-raisin coleslaw: Prepare orange salad dressing, put plumped dark seedless raisins into a bowl, and pour in dressing to cover. Chill raisins and remaining dressing. In a salad bowl, toss desired amounts of shredded carrot and cabbage with the marinated raisins and dressing to coat.

Yield: 6 to 8 servings

Sour Cream Substitute

2 tablespoons skim milk
1 tablespoon lemon juice

1 cup low-fat cottage
 cheese

Mix all ingredients together in a blender at medium-high speed.

Yield: 1 cup

Garlic Dressing

This dressing is excellent with steamed vegetables.

*1 teaspoon mashed
    garlic
1 teaspoon oil*

*1½ tablespoons white wine
    vinegar or lemon juice
    or lime juice*

Warm ingedients over a low heat for 5 minutes.
    If desired, add herbs for more flavor (oregano, rosemary, dill, etc.).

Yield: 2 tablespoons

Ginger Dressing for Chicken

*2 tablespoons olive oil
1 tablespoon cider vinegar
2 teaspoons powdered
    ginger*

*1 teaspoon soy sauce
1 teaspoon mashed garlic
1 tablespoon sesame seeds
    (may be browned)*

Mix all ingredients together in blender.

Yield: 4 tablespoons

French Dressing #1

*Juice of 1 large lemon
1 medium onion, finely
    chopped
1 cup catsup*

*2 cups olive oil
2 tablespoons apple cider
    vinegar
¾ cup granulated sugar*

Mix very well with beater. Keep refrigerated.

Yield: 4 cups

French Dressing #2

1 cup catsup
1 cup olive oil
¾ cup granulated sugar

1 clove garlic, crushed
¼ cup cider vinegar
½ teaspoon paprika

Mix or beat together until smooth. Keep refrigerated.

Yield: 3 cups

Lo-Cal Dressing

1 cup tomato juice
¼ cup lemon juice (or oil)

Herbs to taste
Pinch of sugar sweetener

Shake well; keep refrigerated.

Yield: 1¼ cups

Spicy Lo-cal Dressing

1 cup skim milk
Lemon pepper
¼ teaspoon dry mustard in
  1 tablespoon water
1 teaspoon Worcestershire
  sauce

Dash cayenne pepper
1 tablespoon vinegar
1 clove garlic, crushed
Pinch sweetener

Mix thoroughly and refrigerate.
  This is good on salad, also leftover fish.

Yield: 1 cup

Pine Nut Dressing

This dressing would be delicious tossed with spinach greens.

½ cup chopped pine nuts
¼ cup olive oil
3 tablespoons tarragon
  vinegar

¼ teaspoon grated lemon
  peel
½ teaspoon salt
Dash nutmeg

Combine all ingredients.

Yield: ¾ cup (good for 1½ quarts of greens)

Lime-Cherry Dressing

⅓ cup fresh lime juice
½ cup olive oil
¼ teaspoon salt

⅛ teaspoon paprika
3 tablespoons maraschino
  cherry sryup

Put all ingredients into blender container. Cover and process at medium speed until well mixed. Serve over fruit or vegetable salads.

Yield: about ¾ cup

Walnut Dressing

2 ounces shelled walnuts,
  chopped
2 teaspoons lime juice

2 teaspoons granulated sugar
Generous ½ cup low-fat
  plain yogurt

Chop walnuts.

In a small bowl, beat together lime juice, chopped walnuts, sugar, and yogurt.

Delicious with 4 medium carrots, shredded, and 2 apples, peeled and shredded.

Yield: about ¾ cup

Papaya Seed Dressing

½ cup sugar
2 teaspoons salt
½ teaspoon dry mustard
½ cup white vinegar

½ cup olive oil
½ cup chopped onion
2 tablespoons fresh papaya
seeds

Place all ingredients except papaya seeds into blender or food processor fitted with the metal blade. Blend; add papaya seeds and process only until they are the size of coarsely ground black pepper.

The dressing may be refrigerated up to 3 days.

It is delicious with: 2 heads romaine lettuce, 1 head bibb lettuce, 1 papaya (peeled and sliced), and 1 large avocado (peeled and sliced).

Yield: 12 servings

Yogurt Dressing

1 cup low-fat plain yogurt
1½ to 2 tablespoons lemon
juice

½ teaspoon cinnamon
1 to 2 tablespoons honey
or brown sugar

Stir and add honey or sugar to taste.

Good with apples, dates, and hazelnuts on lettuce.

Yield: about 1 cup

FRUIT DISHES

Fruit makes excellent light desserts and light meals, especially in summer. The added fiber makes fruit a year-round plus for your diet.

Tapioca Stewed Fruit

¼ cup pearl tapioca
⅔ cup water
1 8-ounce package mixed dried fruit or 8 ounces dried peaches, apricots, and pears, mixed
½ cup coarsely chopped dried apples
½ cup coarsely chopped pitted prunes
¼ cup currants

¼ cup chopped fresh cranberries
2 cups water
2 cups apricot nectar
½ cup packed brown sugar
½ orange, sliced thinly, seeds removed
½ lemon, sliced thinly, seeds removed
1 cinnamon stick

Soak pearl tapioca in water overnight. Add remaining ingredients. Pour into 3-quart casserole or Dutch oven; cover. Bake at 350° for 65 to 75 minutes, until thickened and fruit is soft. Remove from oven; let set until cool enough to eat. Remove cinnamon stick. Serve warm or refrigerate and serve cold.

Yield: 6 servings

Prunes with Fruit

In 2-quart pan boil 1 cup water with ½ cup sugar, stirring until sugar dissolves. Add 18 pitted prunes and 1 lemon, thinly sliced. Cook slowly 1 minute, covered. Add ½ cup orange-flavored liqueur or orange juice. Cover and let stand at room temperature at least 3 hours. Discard lemon slices or leave in. Can be kept chilled 1 week.

Yield: about 4 servings

Apricot Balls

1 cup dried apricots
½ cup walnuts
½ cup shredded coconut
2 tablespoons wheat germ

4 tablespoons orange juice
⅓ cup finely chopped walnuts

Put apricots, ½ cup walnuts, and coconut through food processor or blender. Add wheat germ and orange juice; mix well. Form into 1-inch balls. Roll in chopped walnuts. Refrigerate.

Yield: 20 to 24 balls

Strawberries Cardinal

1½ quarts fresh strawberries
⅓ cup granulated sugar
1 10-ounce package frozen raspberries, thawed

2 tablespoons granulated sugar
1 tablespoon orange liqueur
1 teaspoon fresh lemon juice

Wash and drain strawberries. Slice if you wish and sprinkle them with the sugar. Toss, cover, and chill. In blender, blend raspberries, 2 tablespoons sugar, orange liqueur, and lemon juice. Cover and chill. Just before serving, ladle sauce over strawberries.

Yield: 8 servings

Fried Apples

4 to 6 apples (Delicious
  apples or any juice
  apples)

⅓ cup olive oil
¼ cup brown sugar

Wash and core apples. Cut into medium-sized slices. Place in skillet, cover, and cook very slowly. After 3 minutes, add sugar. (You may use sugar substitute—¼ to ½ teaspoon—instead of sugar, if you choose. Brown sugar, however, adds flavor.)

Add cinnamon and/or nutmeg if desired.

Watch carefully. Remove cover to thicken juices during the last 2 or 3 minutes of cooking.

Yield: 6 servings

Fruit Salad

2 tablespoons lemon juice
1 20-ounce can pineapple
  chunks in their juice

2 tablespoons cornstarch
3 bananas, sliced
6 oranges, sliced

Mix lemon juice and pineapple juice with cornstarch. Cook until thick; keep stirring slowly. Cool. Stir in bananas first and then add pineapple. Add sliced oranges last.

Yield: 4 servings

DESSERTS

Desserts evolved as rewards to children for eating well. Adults deserve rewards too! These recipes are compatible with your new dietary commitment.

Apple Cake

Fill a 9 × 13 × 2-inch pan with apples (about 5 pounds of Granny Smith or Greenlings), cored, peeled, and sliced thinly.
Sprinkle cinnamon on apples.
Mix 2 tablespoons cornstarch with 1 cup sugar and sprinkle through apples. Mix in with a fork.
Mix in separate bowl:

1 cup flour   *½ pound butter*
¾ to 1 cup brown sugar   *1 package butterscotch*
1 cup uncooked oatmeal   *pudding*

Mix with fork and knife to make a crumb mixture. Cover apples with the preceding mixture.
Bake 30 to 45 minutes at 375°. Check apples for doneness.

Yield: 12 servings

Fruit Cobbler

5 cups peaches, sliced
5 cups blueberries
1 cup dark brown sugar,
  lightly packed
¾ cup flour
¾ cup uncooked quick-
  cooking oatmeal

½ cup butter at room
  temperature
½ teaspoon cinnamon
Pinch salt

Place fruit, mixed, in a 3-quart casserole. Mix other ingredients to form crumbs. Place crumbs on top of fruit and bake 1 hour at 350°.

Yield: 8 servings

Whole-Wheat Cobbler Bars

½ cup honey or brown sugar   *⅓ cup butter*

Beat together.

1¼ cups each whole-wheat
  flour and regular rolled
  oats

½ cup chopped nuts
2 tablespoons sesame seeds
½ teaspoon salt and soda

Mix until crumbly.

Slowly combine both mixtures thoroughly. Press half the mixture into a greased pan about 9 inches square.

Spread with fruit filling (see below); then crumble remaining mixture over top.

Bake in 350° oven about 25 or 30 minutes. Cut into 16 bars.

Yield: 16 servings

Date Filling

8 ounces chopped dates   *¾ cup water*

Slowly simmer about 10 minutes, covered. Stir to thicken.

Apricot Filling

6 ounces dried apricots   *1 cup water*

Slowly simmer about 20 minutes; stir to thicken and add 3 tablespoons honey or brown sugar.

Other fillings such as prunes and raisins can be used.

PART IV

The Challenge: Thriving Versus Surviving

CHAPTER
13 How to Lose Weight Naturally

All arthritis experts agree on one thing: People who have arthritis should not be overweight. You know for yourself that the weight-bearing joints—the knees, hips, and ankles—hurt more and restrict your activity more if you're overweight. What you learn by experience and can see from intuition every expert confirms.

Excessive weight aggravates the nonweight-bearing joints as well. In fact, the entire arthritic condition goes into a downward spiral. How does this painful pattern start in the first place?

As arthritis gets started, activity decreases and anxiety increases. Increasing anxiety in the face of decreasing activity usually leads to frustration. And many of us relieve our frustration by eating snacks and high-calorie foods. Obviously, eating adds weight. But, the weight accumulates almost before we know it because of the decreased activity. What's worse, is that the excessive weight makes the arthritis more intense, and the cycle of overeating and underexercising continues.

To add insult to injury, arthritis makes cooking more difficult. Let's face it, aching hands aren't able to manipulate pots and pans, and standing over a stove brings aches to sore knees. It's easier to eat convenience foods, which are more fattening than the foods I recommend.

THE DOWNWARD SPIRAL

I reluctantly illustrate this situation with an example so you will benefit by learning what not to do.

Lisa asked me for my diet. She is a beautiful young woman of 28. She is on the downward spiral. I told her she would have to follow the diet plan to gain arthritis relief. If she could control the amount of food she ate, she would lose weight at a slow, steady rate. She had been on and off many weight-loss diets, so I was skeptical of her ability to persevere.

Some months later I was a guest speaker in Philadelphia, where I spoke on weight loss and a special liquid-formula diet. Lisa gave me the following note written on the large envelope in which her diet had been sent:

Dr. Scala,

You sent me your arthritis diet plan in this envelope before but I haven't been able to eliminate the bad foods. I like meat and eggs too much. Also, too many desserts.

Would you put me on the 12-week Slimming Diet you described? I think I can stick with it for twelve weeks easily because I once went on liquid protein for five full months without eating. I am now more than 100 pounds overweight.

Lisa speaks for the desperation of many people. First her note tells us and her appearance confirmed that she has tried a fad "liquid protein" diet. This same diet was so dangerous the Food and Drug Administration put an end to it after seventeen people who followed it died. More, even though Lisa survived the diet and lost weight, she regained it and probably more. Then, she didn't have the willpower to stick with a safe diet that is effective for her arthritis and easily helps her to lose her weight.

Fad or quick weight-loss diets are like running away. As Plato said, "you must take yourself with you." Recent research clearly indicates that quick weight loss followed by regaining weight makes it much harder to lose weight the next time. In short, the body adapts to calorie deprivation and protects itself. Lisa was still the same person after the fad diet with the same poor habits and the same lack of self-discipline. But now she has an additional problem—arthritis—and to save herself from a life of anxiety, depression, and severe obesity, she's got to take control.

SUPREME FRUSTRATION

Two of the most frustrating things people can do is look to fashion models for an image to achieve, or look up their weight on a height and weight chart. Let me explain.

DON'T BE TRAPPED BY ADVERTISING

Fashion models have gotten taller and thinner for their heights as this century has progressed. The reasons are obvious; magazine photographs and TV screen tend to make people look heavier than they are. Because these are the major means of advertising communication, it follows that the merchants want their wares to look best, so they use tall, skinny models. The average weight of the consumer has continued to increase. In short, the image is moving further and further from reality. That's built-in anxiety.

WEIGHT CHARTS ARE ONLY A GUIDE

In stark contrast to the fashion image are the weight and height charts compiled from life insurance statistics. They express an "ideal" weight as a function of height, and are based on statistics that analyze who lives longest. They are no more than a guide.

Charts that show average weight and height are somewhat more reasonable, but very few people are average. And statistical tables are usually printed some years after the data have been collected. By then, the social structure has changed even more.

Still more charts require you to decide whether you've got a small, medium, or large frame to go from there. That works, but too often we may have broad hips, but narrow shoulders, and so on. No person is simply one single type.

MORE PRECISE TESTS

Still other methods use a "pinch" test combined with weight to determine body fat composition and use that as an index. This is much more precise, albeit somewhat impractical for most people to calculate. And if that's not bad enough, some experts claim that our body fat content is a sort of "set point" that we subconsciously strive to maintain.

In recent years the determination of body fat has become more routine. At first it was determined by being weighed on a scale and then being weighed while underwater. Because fat floats, it's not hard to determine your body fat content. But weighing in and out of water is inconvenient; there's a better way.

Some doctors and clinics now have a device that they can

put to your body at various places and determine your body fat content.

Once you know your body fat content you can get at an ideal weight quite quickly. I'll use an example.

Chris is 143 pounds and the doctor determined that she is 29% body fat. A good body fat content is about 22%, for women and 15% for men. Therefore she can drop about 5% of her weight to achieve a good target of 22% body fat. That means Chris can reduce by 10 pounds and get down to 133 pounds. She should be able to accomplish this weight loss in less than a month. And no matter what the height/weight charts tell her, that weight would be sound. The remainder of her weight would be what we call lean body mass, which consists of muscle, structural protein, and so on.

A REALISTIC TARGET

A realistic target doesn't have to be expressed in pounds, but may be expressed in terms of your build, body type, and bones. It's fun to turn your old excuses into challenges, so let's go through it.

TOOLS

You'll need a tape measure and a well-lighted room (preferably a bedroom) with a large mirror, where you can be alone. Bring your food diary notebook and a pencil.

Get all your tools, close the door, and strip to your underwear. You can put on a tight bathing suit if you prefer.

MEASUREMENT FIRST

Measure your hips and your waist. Divide the number of inches for your hips into the number for your waist. The ideal results would be about 0.9 for men and about 0.8 for women. Make a note of your actual results.

USE THE MIRROR

Stand facing the mirror. Place hands on hips and find the tops of your hip bones. About 1 inch on each side midway to your crotch is the maximum width you should be. If you're wider, note that you have got to work on getting it narrowed. Because you took the measurement, you can monitor your progress.

Now with your feet together, look at your knees. Do you see a crack of light showing through above and below your knees? If you do, great—if you don't, then note that you've got to narrow those thighs down.

Now look at your neck—do you have a neck? A long slender neck tells you that you are a "longi-type" and can have well-squared shoulders without them being rounded and "beefy." If you have no visible neck, you are a "brachotype" and will always have a broad, heavy upper body.

Look now at your stomach—from just below your breasts (for men and women) to above your crotch. Is it flat, or does it hang out like a huge bulbous mass of flesh? It is probably something in-between. In fact, you've got your measurements to tell you.

Now turn sideways. Look again at the stomach. Is it flat or do you look pregnant? There is no reason why it shouldn't be relatively flat with a slight rounded appearance if your neck is not slender. Men usually fail this test more than women, because a male paunch is accepted in our society when it shouldn't be.

While standing sideways look at your chest. Not withstanding the breasts, which may be large, you can get a feeling for firmness whether you're a man or a woman. Is there a fold of fat around the ribs just above the level of the elbow? Do the breasts carry excess fat? (Don't confuse sagging with fat.) Note these things because they will be the measure of your success in losing weight.

Now look at your buttocks. Squeeze them; are they firm? Poke them, tease them by making a muscle, and squeeze them again. If they are soft at all times, you've got some weight to lose. Make a note.

Use the tape to measure around your thighs, your upper arms, and your chest. Write these measurements in your notebook.

A FINAL ASSESSMENT

Stand in front of the mirror one more time and slowly look at the body you see. Is it, in your opinion, about right—cracks of light above and below the knees, waist 10 to 20% less than hips, long neck or no neck?

After asking these specific questions, make a general assessment. Is the body you see fat? If so, how fat—a lot, soft fat, or just somewhat overweight? Don't be concerned about firmness at this point; just attempt to decide on fatness.

For example, if you're a man of about 40, and have a "gut," which from the side suggests you might be ready to give birth, you're fat! But if you're a 40-year-old woman and your waist measurement is about the same as your hip measurement, you should lose some weight, but it's not serious. If you know you've got to drop a lot of weight, however, then you'd better get serious.

Now weigh yourself and record it in your food diary, because starting now, you're going to begin getting the weight off.

HOW TO GAUGE SUCCESS

From our little exercise in the last section you have a number of parameters that will record success. You can be very precise and weigh yourself and use the tape measure regularly, or simply stand in front of the mirror—and make a general assessment. Don't become bogged down in looking for precise results quickly. Your excess pounds went on slowly, but they can come off evenly and regularly if you work at it consistently, and I'm going to tell you how simply and easily. But first, let's see how it all happens.

HOW WEIGHT LOSS WORKS

Your body obeys the physical laws of the universe, and the most important of those laws—the second law of thermodynamics—dictates what we must do to lose weight. To lose weight you must burn more energy than you consume. You consume energy as food and expend energy by living—by doing normal activities and exercises.

To elaborate on this, your basal metabolic weight each day consumes about 10 calories for each pound of body weight; the normal functions of life require about another 2 calories for each pound and, if you are at all active, you will burn another 1 calorie for each pound. If you exercise as I recommend in Chapter 14, you will burn another 200 calories or more if you persevere.

Suppose you weigh 135 pounds. That translates to 1,350 calories of basal metabolism and 270 for other activities, with

135 for your work. Add 200 for 30 minutes of brisk walking and it totals 1,955 calories. If you reduce your food intake to 800 calories, you will create a deficit of 1,155 calories each day. Because a pound of fat represents about 3,500 calories, you could lose a pound every three or four days. If you followed that plan for four days each week and ate moderately on the other three days, you would lose 10 pounds in as many weeks.

But, you have an added advantage; this diet is designed to make weight loss easy—in fact, painless—so let's get on with the task.

USE YOUR FOOD DIARY

Weight loss is the simplest dietary objective anyone can pursue because it requires only common sense. Keep track of everything you eat, how much, when, and why. Check that you are using *Do* foods. They will bring your weight down at an acceptable rate.

Although this diet increases fiber and decreases fat, you'll need a few special weight loss *Do's* and *Don'ts*.

DO'S FOR WEIGHT LOSS

Do eat for bulk. Eating for bulk is commonsense eating—compare the pat of butter (about 1 ounce), which contains 250 calories to a head of lettuce, or a very large apple, which contains as much as 150 calories. Then throw in another large raw carrot for an additional 100 calories. You could swallow the pat of butter (like chocolate) without even chewing, but not the apple, lettuce, or the carrot. That's what bulk is all about.

Do eat broiled or barbequed chicken (no skin), fish, or other poultry and game.

Do eat starchy foods such as rice, baked potato (no butter or sour cream), or pasta; use plain tomato sauce or a light clam sauce. Eat single servings, no seconds.

Do eat all the green salad you want; if you've learned that tomatoes are not for you, then use zucchini or other vegetables—apples are also excellent. Eat as much of these things as you can.

Do eat foods from the basic recipes, including bran muffins.

Do snack on popcorn, preferably popped in the microwave in a plain paper bag; use very light salt—no butter! For something different, sprinkle Parmesan cheese on it.

Do drink one 8- to 12-ounce glass of water before each meal and preferably eat a fiber snack or bran muffin with it.

Do eat pasta using only simple sauces, not meat sauces. Be sure that the sauces are prepared with generous amounts of vegetables.

Do stick to your supplement program. In fact, you could increase it a little to be on the safe side.

DON'TS FOR WEIGHT LOSS

Don't eat desserts that are not also acceptable for regular meals. Now you know that means no cake, no pie, no pudding, and so on. But you can eat fruit of any kind and any of the gelatin-type salads.

Don't eat vegetables or entrées cooked in oil—even olive oil—more than twice each week.

Don't eat nuts.

HOW IT WILL COME OFF

Weight will come off steadily 1 to 2 pounds per week, if you follow the rules for weight loss. Expect a large surge of weight loss during the first week. Then the weight will drop slowly because you will genuinely be losing body fat and not simply losing water or carbohydrate reserves. When you achieve the realistic figure you deserve, just go back to the basic *Do's, Don'ts*, and *Occasionally's* and the weight will stay off.

In the beginning you might experience a slightly larger surge of weight loss—up to 3% of your body weight within a week—which will be due to water loss. On this diet the water loss will probably be associated with a shift in electrolyte reserves, sodium, and potassium. Don't be surprised if a week or two later you appear to lose weight very slowly or even gain back a pound. It will only be this fluid balance restoring itself; stick with it and you will succeed.

FAD OR STARVATION DIETS

Anyone with arthritis who is willing to make the serious commitment this book represents should not put herself or himself on "magic" or "starvation" diets. They often achieve quick results, but they don't last.

Fad diets work in the short term because they usually restrict calories to less than 800 daily for the first week or two. Under these conditions the body's carbohydrate reserves are often used in the first week or ten days. Because each pound of carbohydrate carries 3 pounds of water, you lose a lot of water quickly. But as your system stabilizes, the carbohydrate reserves are restored along with the water it requires, so the weight loss slows, even stops, or you regain slightly. Then the weight starts coming off again.

The real weight loss on a fad diet of less than 800 calories is just slightly more than on this diet—about ½ pound weekly. But, in exchange for the extra half pound, you run more than one health risk, do nothing for your long-term commitment, and must drink some type of "mulch" to the exclusion of food. How long can you do that?

CONVENIENCE MEAL SUBSTITUTE

Slim-plan products and meal substitutes are for sale in any supermarket or by the distributors of Shaklee products. These products can be used very effectively if you exercise common sense.

First, the meal substitute should contain from 200 to 250 calories for each meal. It should provide 20 grams of protein and 25 to 35% of the U.S. RDA for the nineteen vitamins and minerals. If they mix with skim milk, they will provide more calcium from the milk.

Second, it should contain only 1 or 2 grams of milk fat and no corn oil. Preferably it should be made without nonfat dry milk, but these products are not widely available and often have an unpleasant taste.

Third, if it is to be mixed with milk, you should use only skim milk. Ideally it is made to be mixed with water.

The best way to use these products is to substitute one or two meals daily. Snack on high-fiber products and eat a third meal from the *Do* list. Then stick to the remainder of the extra weight loss *Do's* and *Don'ts*.

CHAPTER
14 Exercise:
The Miracle Drug

Exercise is synergistic. Synergism, from the Greeks, means the sum is greater than its parts. Simply put, if you add the benefits of exercise to your diet, you get something even greater than you might expect.

Whenever you increase your activity, you notice your heart beating faster, which is a major objective of exercise. Think of it as nutrition in which you are dealing with the most important of all the nutrients—oxygen. We can go without food, vitamins, and minerals for months; we can go without water for weeks, but we can go without oxygen for only a few minutes at most. It's that important.

Oxygen, similar to all nutrients, is delivered to the tissues by the blood. When we increase our blood flow, we deliver nourishing oxygen more rapidly and efficiently to every tissue. As our muscle tone improves from exercise, more blood capillaries develop and the entire process becomes more efficient. Unfortunately, the converse of that is also true.

More important, exercise delivers oxygen and other nutrients to the tissues where the movement is taking place, because that is the location of most active metabolism.

It follows that if we flex and move our joints, it will increase the blood flow to them and the surrounding tissues.

This helps to promote healing and restoration of any tissues damaged by arthritis and diminished by inactivity.

Increased blood flow also delivers more oxygen to the brain. This helps us to be more alert, overcome stress, reduce levels of anxiety and depression, and gain a better, more positive outlook. In fact, research has indicated that exercise helps the body to produce materials that chemists call the endorphins. Endorphins act as natural "mood" elevators. In short, exercise done regularly improves the entire being— mentally and physically.

BENEFITS OF FLEXING JOINTS

An old saying teaches that "if you don't use it, you lose it." Do you believe the author had arthritic joints in mind? I do!

By moving and working the joints—all of them—we increase flexibility. Exercise reduces, if not stops and in many cases reverses the insidious crippling that comes with rheumatoid arthritis. At the very least, exercise preserves joint mobility. The benefits can be enormous and require as little as 15 minutes twice each day—a small investment with great rewards.

MUSCLE TONE—STRENGTH AND APPEARANCE

Exercise directly involves the muscles and they benefit most. Muscles increase in strength, general tone, and capacity for exercise. This provides increased reserve capacity by helping them to become larger. Experts say that exercise builds lean body mass. Muscle is lean tissue; it contains very little fat.

Muscles are generally smooth in appearance. Consequently, as your muscle mass increases, appearance generally improves. Lumpy fat disappears.

Daily tasks will become easier as your reserve capacity increases. You are kin to the athlete who trains for an event by practicing beyond the demands of the event.

WEIGHT

By increasing your energy output regularly, the calories you burn will accumulate, and by controlling your food intake, your weight will slowly decrease. More important, your dimensions will improve because of the benefits I've already described as "muscle tone." In fact, very often people don't really need to lose weight. They simply need to transfer the calories they store and carry around as lumpy fat into lean muscle. In the twentieth century, and our land of plenty, there's no need to carry a paunch as a reserve for times of scarcity; it's seen as ugly fat!

A LITTLE ARITHMETIC

Never rely on exercise as the only means to lose weight. For example, 1 pound of body fat represents 3,500 extra calories. If you exercise faithfully, doing both limbering exercises and calorie-burning exercises (such as walking), you could burn about 200 calories each day. At that rate you would lose only 1 pound in seventeen days. But, good news if you do it, each pound will seem like three in appearance.

By dieting and exercising, you can increase your calorie deficit to 500 each day without really trying. For example, by simply stopping snacks and desserts the combination of diet and exercise will, on average, take off a pound every seven days! If that doesn't seem fast enough, simply follow the advice in Chapter 13 and you can easily increase that by over 50% to 1½ pounds every seven days.

BENEFITS OF MORE MUSCLE

If the appearance of increased muscle mass isn't incentive enough, the physical advantage in movement and feeling is even better. But, you'll never feel the most important advantages—increased basal metabolic rate. Basal metabolism is the energy your body spends to keep things running. For example, even while you sleep your heart is beating, your lungs are extracting oxygen from the air, kidneys are constantly removing wastes from your blood—even your brain is sifting and cataloging the day's information—each organ is active; there's a lot going on. Nutritionists call this activity the basal metabolism. Basal metabolism accounts for the majority of calories we burn each 24 hour day.

FAT IS DORMANT

Now if you think of fat as "dormant" tissue, it uses an absolute minimum of the body's energy. After all, fat is storage energy, and God made it for times of scarcity so during times of plenty it would require only miniscule energy for maintenance. That's why a fat body has a much lower metabolic rate than a lean body.

Another thing to consider is that much human fat is located just beneath the skin, where it serves as a layer of insulation. This insulating layer of fat keeps body heat in and conserves the energy required to maintain body temperature. This insulation also helps to reduce the basal metabolic rate in fat people.

Lean muscle is anything but dormant. It is packed with blood capillaries and even stores its own energy as a carbohydrate called glycogen. You might say God recognized that muscles would need quick energy and couldn't bother with mobilizing fat reserves in times of need.

UNEXPECTED BENEFITS

Satisfaction comes with accomplishment; we humans respond to positive reinforcement. You will begin to find satisfaction as you gain flexibility, shift fat to muscle, and can perform tasks you had once thought hopeless. But that's no different than doing anything well.

Mental alertness always improves because improved muscle tone brings improved circulation. It follows that improved circulation brings more oxygen and nourishment to your master organ—the brain.

Sleep will be sounder, not because you are tired; on the contrary you will have more energy. You sleep better because everything about your body is more efficient. And although the restrictive power of sound sleep remains a scientific mystery, no one can ever doubt its miraculous value, both mental and physical.

Regularity of bowel function will improve, another of the synergistic benefits of exercise with your dietary commitment. Although dietary fiber improves regularity and bowel function, the regularity of exercise, which tones all muscles, including those of the bowel, helps them to respond easily and regularly.

Bone strength will also increase. A national epidemic of osteoporosis is sweeping the United States. Osteoporosis is a decline in bone density due in large part to inadequate dietary calcium and exercise in the childhood and adolescent years. Once women are past the menopause, hormonal changes bring about an acceleration of bone loss, so it is even more critical. Two factors require personal control—dietary calcium and exercise. This dietary plan will take care of the calcium but only you can take care of the exercise.

NEVER TOO OLD

Dr. Anthony Albanese once conducted a study on post-menopausal women. He supplemented their diets with calcium and had them engage in a very modest exercise program, such as walking. In every case the women showed a significant increase in bone density as precisely measured by x-ray methods. More important, their energy increased, they felt better, and they became more active. None of this would be either surprising or even important if the women didn't average 82 years in age! They proved that no one is ever too old to improve.

Age brings wisdom and efficiency to the body; your basal metabolism actually declines with age. It also brings a decline in physiological capacity. Therefore your physical capacity is limited and any exercise should be similarly limited. In other words, don't go beyond your limits, but don't underestimate your limits.

AN EXERCISE PROGRAM

Arthritis Relief Beyond Drugs, written by Rachel Carr, contains a complete system of muscle flexing, stretching, and limbering exercises for people with arthritis. These exercises are beautifully explained and illustrated. I urge you to obtain this inexpensive book and follow its programs. But I will review some salient exercises for you here.

FIFTEEN MINUTES TWICE A DAY

Basic limbering, stretching and breathing exercises should be done twice daily and should take less than 15 minutes each time. As you become more involved with them, don't allow the 15 minutes to decline to 10 minutes; instead, increase the amount of each.

BASIC BREATHING EXERCISES

Our objective here is to strengthen the lungs and improve on their ability to extract oxygen from the air. This is basic to our mental and physical well-being.

Abdominal breathing is best done lying down; it requires you to hold your chest still and breathe by expanding your abdomen. It is done by breathing in for a long five count and breathing out for a long five count. Repeat this twice daily about five times or more, and you will realize it helps you relax.

Chest breathing can be done standing, and requires expanding the rib cage on a long five count as you breathe in and then exhaling on a long five count. This can be practiced anytime and should be done frequently.

STRETCHING-FLEXING

Lower Back

Lower-back stretching is done by simply lying on your back (do after deep breathing), and raising your knees with your hands interlocked on your abdomen. Tighten your buttocks and pull down on your abdomen so your lower back touches the floor. Repeat this ten times.

Spinal Stretch

Kneel down with arms on floor, slide your arms forward until your head touches the floor. Keep your hips above the knees with your tocs on the floor (still kneeling). Then slide back to the original kneeling position with your hips (buttocks) resting on your heels.

Pelvic Stretch

This exercise is difficult, but much is gained if you only try. If you keep trying you will eventually be able to do it, and that is a sure sign of progress. Lie on your back with your feet flat on the floor (knees bent). Then with your arms flat on the floor at your sides, raise your buttocks so you shift your weight to your shoulders and feet. This should be done five times, no matter how little you can raise your buttocks.

Sit-ups

Everyone hates sit-ups, but hang in there for a few minutes. I don't care if you only start with one-half of one. Do it! It will strengthen your back and abdominal muscles.

Lie on your back, hands behind head, knees bent, and sit up. If you can't make it, go as far as you can—call it a "head-up." It will gradually strengthen the muscles of your back and abdomen. Aim for five and keep working toward twenty-five over time.

Back Leg Raises

Lying on your stomach, clasp hands behind back. Keep legs tight, raise your chest and legs at the same time so your back is arched. Even if you only get your feet and head up at first, this is excellent for the back muscles and the spine. Work toward ten daily.

Stand Up Lunge

This is easy and it's great for knees, hips, and ankles. Put right hand on right hip; holding right leg in place, take a giant step, place left hand on left knee and bend as far forward as possible, holding right foot in place and right hand on right hip. You'll either feel like a dancer, fencer, explorer, or just plain foolish.

Do this exercise at least five times on each leg. In fact, you can do it anytime you wish; it limbers knees, hips, and ankles. You see runners do it before a distance run so it must be effective.

Knee Bends

Two types of knee bends are for us. Sit in a straight chair. Alternately raise one leg to the horizontal and hold it for a slow five count. Do five to ten for each leg and each time increase a little in either time or number. You can do this one whenever you sit in a chair.

A second knee bend is easy and requires you to sit on the floor. As you sit on the floor with legs out, bring left foot on top of right leg and pull with hands as high as possible, so you're half cross-legged. Do it five times with each leg. This is excellent for the knees.

Hip Strength

Stand straight; arms at sides. Now keeping legs straight, looking forward, bend to the right, keeping arm at side. Get arm as low as possible down the leg. Do it five times on each side, attempting to reach the floor with your hand.

Hip Rotation

Hold something moderately heavy in your hands at waist level while standing tall. The telephone book is excellent; this book is probably too light. Now simply hold it in your hands and rotate as far to each side as possible, holding it at each side for a slow five count. You can do this exercise any time of the day anywhere; it's easy, not strenuous, and will do much good.

Shoulder Rotation

Place hands on same shoulders and raise your elbows horizontal with shoulders. While horizontal, rotate forward so your elbows are in front of your face. Touch elbows. Now raise your elbows over your head with hands still on shoulders.

Repeat this entire sequence as often as you wish, but do it at least five times. It is another of those stretches that can be done as often as you wish, any time of day.

Now put hands at sides and rotate first one shoulder, then the other. Then clasp hands in back and repeat your shoulder rotation. You cannot do this too often.

Towel Stretch

With a small towel (dish size), hold towel with left hand outstretched and pull with the right hand. Alternate hands. While pulling, put as much strength into the pull as possible.

Then take the towel, hang it over your left shoulder with left hand, and grip with right hand from right side around your back. Pull moderately hard, left hand against right hand. Do this five times alternating.

Hand Exercises

Arthritis is unmerciful to the joints of the hands. It can restrict their mobility to less than 10% and deform them even more. But don't lament over what's been lost; resolve to retain what you have and recapture some flexibility that you thought was lost.

Working with hands can be very painful. Go slowly; even if

you only do one half or less at first, persevere. You will find that it slowly increases with each attempt. But don't do any to the point of serious pain.

Hand Stretch–Wrist Rotation

Stretch your hand as far open as possible. If you can place your palm on the table with outstretched fingers higher than the palm, you are in excellent shape. If not, keep trying. If necessary, use the other hand to help stretch; then clench into a fist. Repeat this at least five times for each hand and do it as often as possible throughout the day.

Touch your index finger to the thumb. If necessary, use your other hand to help as much as possible. Then the second finger and so on through the pinky. Do it with each finger until you have a fist, then reverse the process.

Holding your right hand above the wrist with your left hand, rotate your right wrist by bringing your right hand palm up and rotate from left to right, back and forth. *Caution:* If your wrist pains when you do this, go slowly and limit your movement. If you attempt, or complete, five at a time, you will, over the weeks, notice an increase in mobility. This is another exercise that can be done any time.

ASSISTED EXERCISE

In Chapter 21 we will explore the concept of support groups—groups where people get together to discuss self-help and support each other's efforts. Exercise can be a terrific way to help each other. Any of the exercises I've discussed can be done with assistance from someone.

Assisted exercise is an excellent way to get started, especially for joints that are swollen and stiff. You must be cautious in your enthusiasm so you don't injure someone you want to help. Start slowly and cautiously; there's no hurry. It took a long time to get your joints into this shape; it will take time to get them out.

MORE VIGOROUS EXERCISE

Suppose you can breeze through the exercises I've outlined. Fantastic! But do them for 15 minutes twice daily and you are ready for more, and there's a great deal available for you.

My mother is 80 years old; she uses an exercise bicycle in her living room while watching TV. I estimate she uses from 200 to 250 calories each day she does it, which is about four times each week. But she started much more modestly on this diet.

My mother is an excellent example of the ultimate objective of exercise. Do it with moderate vigor for from 20 to 30 minutes or more, depending on type. I use her to illustrate the point that you are never too old. I expect the same effort from her great-grandchildren, who should fast jog about 3 miles. This level of activity will accomplish all those health benefits I described in the beginning of this chapter. And most important are the mental benefits.

TELEVISION STRETCHING

If you are up to it, there are daily TV exercise programs that emphasize stretching and limbering. Many of them are quite advanced and you simply cannot keep up. But get the motion down properly and go at your own pace. Remember, you are not expected to keep up with or exceed what they are doing; rather your pace is determined by your own body. More recently videotapes of slow-paced exercise have become available.

AEROBICS

An aerobics craze is sweeping our nation and it's the best thing that could have happened. Some aerobics instructors conduct classes for people with restricted capability. If there's an aerobics class in your community, see if there's a group you can enter. Sometimes, if you have a group of similarly interested friends (Chapter 21), an instructor will hold a special session.

In addition, some TV stations offer aerobics instruction for people who have physical limitations.

If none of that works, you can purchase records and tapes to accomplish the same thing. That's another advantage of organizing an arthritis self-help group to help search out these facilities.

VIGOROUS WALKING

Once you have done the limbering and stretching exercises, I want you to do them at your own pace daily. Remember there are many others you can do and I only described the basics.

Walking is an excellent exercise. It should be done in comfortable shoes, uninterrupted, with good surroundings and in safe areas. Most important, it should be done for 30 to 40 minutes at each session. If you can walk twice daily, that is great!

Start walking short distances; two blocks is fine. Stop and rest if you need to. Don't hurt your knee joints by overdoing it; simply resolve to start small and work up to bigger and better things.

Walking should be vigorous, so learn to swing your arms as you go. Breathe deeply and consistently. Do it regularly. Set aside some time each day to exercise.

The calories expended in walking range from 5 to about 8 per minute. So 40 minutes of walking ranges from 200 to 320, depending on vigor, terrain, and your weight. As a rule of thumb, you should strive for 250 to 300 calories per session about four or five times each week. That comes back to 40 minutes.

CYCLING

One woman who has followed this plan now cycles regularly; in her words:

Dr. Scala, "I'm so excited; I haven't been able to ride my bicycle for over twenty years."

Her letter expressed such excitement it came right off the paper; that's what life is all about.

Bicycling, at a moderate, safe cycling speed, consumes about 10 calories per minute. Therefore 20 to 30 minutes is excellent. It builds aerobic capacity and there is no pounding on any joints. It's got everything going for it and nothing against it.

Three-wheel bikes are now available for adults, which make this activity possible at any age. In addition, it can become the transportation for shopping, errands, and socializing. It also has tremendous social value because anyone you meet on a bicycle already shares a common interest.

SWIMMING

Swimming is the best exercise of all. It places no stress on joints, it uses most of the muscle groups, and it's fun. To be effective, you should strive for about 30 minutes of nonstop swimming. And it need not be the fast crawl stroke shown on "Wide World of Sports." Just keep moving with a doggie paddle, breaststroke, backstroke, or sidestroke. If you can eventually knife through the water like a sea otter, excellent. You have made my day. Simply be realistic, do it regularly for about 30 minutes, and you will have achieved excellence.

SPORTS ACTIVITIES

Tennis is great, but golf is one way to ruin a good walk. Golf is good for recreation, but is not a means of exercise. There are many recreational sports that have many merits. Think through each one to see whether it provides vigorous activity for 20 to 40 minutes. If it does, then it's excellent; if not, do it for social purposes and exercise at other times.

MECHANICAL BICYCLES AND OTHER DEVICES

Through the marvels of modern engineering you can exercise regularly in the privacy of your home. All of these devices provide exercise with no jarring of joints and bones, complete safety, and convenience. Simply remember that you get what you pay for, and it's better to spend more money for one that will last.

Exercise bicycles emphasize the legs. Get one where you can adjust the tension so your output can reach your capability. The advantage is that you can read, listen to the radio, or watch television while doing it. This helps to fight boredom and can be an educational experience.

Rowing machines are very good because the better ones allow for leg, arm, and hip activity at the same time. They increase upper body tone a little more than lower body, which is good because we tend to use our legs more in daily activity.

Rowing machines use from 10 to 15 calories per minute, so 20 minutes, at low speed, should be the objective.

Nordic Track is, in my opinion, the very best. It is what I use. It stimulates cross-country skiing, which exercises, in a beneficial way, both the upper and lower body. The Nordic Track requires a little practice to get started, but even that will help your coordination. You can adjust both leg resistance and arm resistance so it can be completely individualized for personal capacity and objective. It can be set to consume from 8 to 15 calories per minute, depending on the speed you use.

JOGGING

If you're a jogger, you should already be doing all the proper limbering and stretching exercises. I want you to consider that jogging places stress on all the weight-bearing joints, the back, and even the shoulders. It should be done in moderation by people with arthritis.

AFTERTHOUGHTS

This chapter is by no means comprehensive. There are as many forms of exercise as there are recreational activities. My objective is to get you started on limbering, stretching, and some regular activity. The benefits are so great that it usually gains its own momentum.

I urge everyone to purchase one of the many books on the subject, join a local group, or participate through radio, television, or by video rental.

CHAPTER
15 Your Chance to Control Ulcers

About 13% of people who have rheumatoid arthritis also have ulcers. But worse, some medication used for arthritis relief, such as aspirin, can contribute to ulcer development.

The most recent thinking on ulcer development teaches that there is some involvement of the antagonistic prostaglandins in helping the mucous membranes protect against excess acid. If this hypothesis is correct—and there is no reason to believe it is not—the use of aspirin or other general inhibitors of these metabolic pathways would be a definite aggravating, if not causative influence. This is what is meant by an unwanted side effect.

Our dietary commitment should have a twofold basic beneficial effect on ulcers. It is designed to restore balance to the prostaglandins and not to eliminate even the antagonistic. Using the "tug-of-war" analogy, we only want to get both sides even or give a modest edge to the beneficial. Therefore if aspirin or other aspirin derivatives can be reduced, the ulcer will no longer be favored or aggravated. After that, some commonsense rules and other features of this diet should apply. Any ulcer sufferer should pursue a low-fat, high-carbohydrate diet. This is logical when you recognize that a low-fat carbohydrate-rich diet is more easily digested. It requires a lesser production of stomach acid and helps hasten stomach emptying without an acid rebound. I'd better explain acid rebound.

ACID REBOUND

Normally an empty stomach is on the acid side of neutral. When we eat food or drink a beverage, acid is produced because the food or beverage brings the stomach contents more toward neutral. If the food is not excessive in fat, contains protein and complex carbohydrate, the acid level will be restored to normal as the food digests, and the stomach will empty its contents into the small intestine for complete digestion.

Some things cause the stomach to overshoot its acid target and become more acidic than normal. These include coffee, fat, and nicotine. This acid rebound—excessive acid—can overpower the neutralizing capacity of the small intestine, eventually resulting in an ulcer there. It can also help to erode the stomach lining itself and produce a stomach ulcer.

The lesson is to avoid food and beverages that cause excessive acid production. The beverage of choice is tea because it doesn't cause an acid rebound and it helps speed stomach emptying. Coffee, both regular and decaffeinated, should be avoided. Our dietary commitment is not rich in fat, is adequate in protein, rich in complex carbohydrates and fiber, all of which help produce normal acid production.

HEREDITY

Ulcer sufferers usually produce more acid than average, and antacids are helpful to them in protecting the stomach. Antacids work on a simple principle. They neutralize the acid in the stomach. For example, a reasonable neutralizer is bicarbonate of soda—baking soda. Pour some vinegar (an acid) on some in a bowl and watch it foam as the acid is neutralized and gas (carbon dioxide) is released. The objective is to neutralize stomach acid, but not excessively. To do this use just enough antacid between meals, but eat enough food to keep the stomach working. Don't get in the habit of going around with an empty stomach and constantly using antacids to feel normal. Develop the habit of eating normal meals and not using acidic beverages such as coffee and soft drinks on an empty stomach. Drink hot or iced tea or water.

ALCOHOL AND ULCERS

Alcohol, usually in the form of a predinner cocktail, is taken to "arouse the appetite"; it gets the juices flowing. Stomach juices are acid and contain digestive enzymes. If food is on its way, it's not a problem if drinking continues, but if the food keeps getting put off, the acid continues with nothing to digest except stomach lining. Logic tells you to eat when you drink—and the predinner cocktail should be exactly what it's meant to be—a predinner cocktail!

CHAPTER
16 How to Bring Down High Blood Pressure

If you've got high blood pressure, you're not alone. By the age of 35, 25% of arthritics have this problem; by age 60, 70% have it.

Some of us inherit high blood pressure and others inherit a tendency to develop high blood pressure.

WHAT TO DO ABOUT HEREDITY

Heredity is a convenient excuse. People who complain, "It's in my genes," and do nothing are simply dropping out. If they understood the food-related causes of high blood pressure, they might realize how foolish it is not to make an effort to change their eating habits. Most people go through life frustrated by things they feel they can't change. Don't fall into that trap. Change takes a little extra effort, once you've made the commitment to try.

FOOD-RELATED CAUSES OF HIGH BLOOD PRESSURE

Sodium and potassium are the two major factors to consider. They are involved in the transmission of nerve impulses, but they are also involved in our water balance. In that respect they influence blood pressure.

Sodium is commonly found as salt, which consists essentially of sodium and chloride. One hundred milligrams of salt contain about 50 milligrams of sodium. Sodium is found in body fluids such as blood plasma. Think of it as the mineral that maintains the fluid in between the body's cells.

Potassium in contrast is not obtained naturally as a salt, although potassium salt is prescribed as a supplement for some people taking diuretics for high blood pressure. Potassium is obtained from the food we eat. Potassium is the mineral that maintains the fluid inside our cells.

Our bodies actually contain more potassium than sodium, and an adult requires about 1,800 milligrams of potassium each day compared with about 1,500 milligrams of sodium. People should easily get enough potassium from the food they eat, but many do not. They can increase potassium by using more natural foods.

Americans live in a sea of sodium. The average person consumes from 7 to 10 grams or more of salt daily. That's more than two and usually well over three times as much as they require. But worse, the ratio of potassium to sodium is completely reversed. Instead of getting somewhat more potassium than sodium, we get about three times the sodium as potassium. Obviously that ratio causes a lot of work for the kidneys to restore balance, and in many people it results in high blood pressure.

HOW TO CONTROL SODIUM

My blood pressure is never above 110 over 70; it's in my genes to have low blood pressure. But I strive to keep my salt intake below 3,000 milligrams daily to about 1,800 milligrams or less of sodium. Similarly, I strive to keep my potassium intake at or above the same level—both, in balance. It's easy—simply follow this dietary program.

God made fruits, vegetables, grains, meats, and most natural foods so they contain more potassium than sodium. In short, an ideal balance exists in natural foods, and if we use natural foods as much as possible, select processed foods sensibly, and get rid of the salt shaker, our sodium/potassium balance will be normal. Examine processed foods and see what humans have done.

SODIUM CONTENT OF FOOD

Salt was so scarce 2,000 years ago that Roman soldiers were paid in salt; it was a medium of commerce like gold dust to the forty-niners. In fact, this "salt ration" was eventually reduced to a single word, *salary*, which we all recognize as the paycheck for services rendered. Unfortunately, since Roman times we've learned to harvest salt so effectively we can afford to use it to melt ice off sidewalks.

Man is born with an ability to detect salt—for good reason—survival. An infant drinking salt water will dehydrate and, if not stopped, will die. But our food habits teach us to like salty things; in many, if not all of our snacks that salty taste is prominent. Although this is obvious in such snacks as popcorn, potato chips, and french fries, it is more subtle in other processed food. Salt is found in most processed foods, ranging from a Big Mac to breakfast cereal. Slowly over the years as we grow we develop an affection for salt. Salt is also one of the best natural preservatives and it is used in foods, especially canned goods and meat products, to prevent the growth of microorganisms. In about 1870, however, food technologists began using it to manipulate the taste of processed foods. The outcome of this growth in processed food is that we live in a "sea of salt"—it's everywhere.

THE SALT SEA

A chicken breast has about 40 milligrams of sodium and 220 milligrams of potassium, which is low sodium by any standards, and the potassium/sodium ratio is excellent. But purchase the same chicken breast at a fast-food outlet where it's coated and cooked in grease under high pressure, and it contains 1,200 milligrams of sodium with the same 220 milligrams of potassium—almost all your daily sodium in one part of one meal! Nature's ratio of potassium to sodium is obliterated!

Similarly I could compare the all-American hamburger, which contains about 100 milligrams of sodium and 250 milligrams of potassium when you prepare it on your backyard barbeque. In contrast, the fast-food hamburger usually has about 700 to 800 milligrams of sodium and the same amount of potassium.

Fillet of flounder contains 240 milligrams of sodium and 590 milligrams of potassium per serving. This is an excellent ratio by any standards, and the levels of both are superb; it illustrates another example of why this diet plan is excellent. In contrast, if you purchase the fillet breaded and frozen, the sodium jumps to over 700 milligrams per serving, whereas the potassium remains at 590 milligrams. Not only is the sodium more than doubled, but the ratio of sodium to potassium is reversed. In short, what God provided in nature man has obliterated!

Homemade pancakes made from a standard recipe contain

just under 200 milligrams of sodium per serving and about 60 milligrams of potassium—not great—not bad if your other food is right—it's okay. Mixes such as Aunt Jemima's and Mrs. Smith's contain about 600 milligrams of sodium and about 100 milligrams of potassium—more than three times the sodium and less than double the potassium. Obliterated again!

Breakfast cereals are a lesson in self-control and label reading.

Oatmeal contains 1 milligram of sodium and 100 milligrams of potassium if prepared without adding any salt. Add salt according to directions and it contains 280 milligrams, which I consider excessive. By simply exercising a little control, you can hold that to less than 100 and the taste is better.

All-Bran cereal contains 320 milligrams of sodium and 350 milligrams of potassium, a respectable ratio and not too much sodium even though most people don't know it's there (read the ingredients). But All-Bran provides excellent fiber content, which is its redeeming feature!

Cap'n Crunch—no redeeming features—contains 213 milligrams of sodium and 36 milligrams of potassium. Bad! With no fiber! None!

Cornflakes contains 350 milligrams of sodium and only 26 milligrams of potassium—too much sodium, not enough potassium, and no fiber. Cornflakes and Cap'n Crunch are examples of high-sodium excuses to drink a glass of milk with a cereal spoon! Stupid!

Spinach illustrates nature's balance with 71 milligrams of sodium and 470 milligrams of potassium—super! Canned spinach contains 356 milligrams of sodium and 317 milligrams of potassium. In contrast to canned, frozen is about the same as fresh, so use frozen vegetables if you can't get fresh.

READING FOOD LABELS FOR SODIUM

Not all food products show the sodium and potassium content on the label. You should urge more manufacturers to provide this voluntary labeling service. Therefore you should first look to see whether the information is there; if it is, keep the number 2,500 milligrams in mind. You should attempt to hold your sodium to 2,500 milligrams daily as an absolute upper limit. I prefer under 2,000 milligrams!

If the sodium content is not provided quantitatively, look at the ingredient list. If salt is among the top three ingredients, you should question your need for the product, especially if you have high blood pressure. If it is not among the top five, don't worry about it.

HIGH BLOOD PRESSURE AND THIS DIET

If you follow my advice about sodium and stay with this dietary plan, your blood pressure should slowly come into line if it is high because of weight, sodium, or other dietary factors. With some people it will drop rather quickly, because of the natural low sodium content of the diet and its balance with potassium.

CALCIUM CAN HELP

For a relatively few people, restoration of the RDA in calcium will also help bring blood pressure into line. Because our dietary commitment provides the RDA in calcium either by diet or supplements, it should be adequate.

CHAPTER

17 Beating Anxiety and Depression

Which came first, the chicken or the egg? You should ask the same question about anxiety, depression, and arthritis. All the arthritics I know are or have been anxious about their situation; all experience depression just thinking about their problem. And the younger they are the more anxious they become.

BLOOD SUGAR—KEEP IT LEVEL

Our brain responds to many changes; after all, it's designed to do that for survival. The body's major source and the brain's only source of energy is the blood sugar glucose. It should be no surprise that the brain responds negatively to a drop in blood sugar; it also responds to elevated blood sugar, but we need not be concerned with that here.

A drop in blood sugar can be interpreted in this way: The body is telling the brain that its source of energy is dwindling. If no obvious signs of energy are forthcoming (e.g., eating), the brain starts sending basic signals that show outwardly as irritablity and anxiety. If it remains low, it could lead to a lessened activity, even a feeling of depression.

So the first rule is to maintain a normal blood sugar level. Maintaining good consistent blood sugar means not giving your body a high sugar load, because it responds with an overproduction of insulin. The hormone insulin helps to get sugar into the cells to be metabolized, and an overproduction of insulin will be followed by an excessive decline in blood sugar. This is hypoglycemia, which means low blood sugar. It can happen to a normal person who isn't eating properly, and is not a disease. We should all strive to avoid it, especially people with arthritis.

Maintaining normal blood sugar is easy—avoid a high-sugar load. Stick to complex carbohydrates, which also come with lots of dietary fiber, and maintain a good balanced protein supply. Does that sound familiar? It should; I have designed this dietary commitment to be rich in complex carbohydrates, moderate in fat, and adequate if somewhat high in protein— all of which add up to a stable blood sugar.

The second rule is to avoid large slugs of sugar. Don't eat candy, don't use soft drinks (diet types are okay if you don't have ulcers), and use desserts in moderation or select those that contain fiber, such as fruit, fruit pies, carrot cake, and others.

STIMULANTS

It's hard for people to get used to the idea that caffeine is addictive. That's correct; it is as addictive as nicotine and other narcotics. If you're a coffee drinker, just stop cold turkey for two days and you'll soon know from experience what withdrawal symptoms are like. Caffeine stimulates the central nervous system and excessive amounts can overstimulate and produce erratic activity. Who has not heard of "coffee nerves"?

It follows that what can pick you up and add to anxiety can later let you down and contribute to depression. The Greeks said it all over 3,000 years ago—moderation. Moderation in stimulant use is essential. Stimulants increase both anxiety and depression. One or two cups of coffee daily should be enough.

ALCOHOL

In early stages of drinking, inhibitions loosen so that alcohol acts as a stimulant and conversation catalyst. But as metabolism loses ground to the rate of alcohol intake, the senses begin to dull and depression begins. All this leads to the conclusion that alcohol is a drug that should be taken seriously. It is definitely best to avoid drinking, but second best is to use it in moderation—a glass of wine with a meal or a cocktail before dinner.

POSITIVE THINKING

When I speak on nutrition and stress, people often ask what supplements to take for stress. I tell them that dealing with stress and the anxiety-depression spiral it produces is the same as preparing for an athletic event. However it's not as simple or as obvious.

We prepare for an athletic event or other performance by practicing. Nutrition is essential because it helps us to practice longer, harder, and more efficiently; it's the foundation of good health. Similarly with mental health, but with a subtle difference. I can't help you practice for stress; only you can do that. That's where the concept of a positive, motivated attitude comes in; that's the practice, and you have to do it all the time. We'll explore the concepts and some simple approaches that can help in Chapter 20.

NUTRIENTS, ANXIETY, AND DEPRESSION

I hope you realize that anxiety and depression management requires good nutrition to keep blood sugar constant, together with moderation in common drugs like caffeine and alcohol. The metabolism of blood sugar and alcohol is dependent on a sound nutritional foundation. That includes all the vitamins and minerals, especially the B vitamins and the minerals zinc, magnesium, and iron.

Therefore be sure you get enough of these to satisfy your own personal needs. You've got to keep in touch with how you feel and make sure your nutritional foundation is sound. Remember, you are an individual different from everyone else. Consequently you might require more than your neighbor —or you might require less.

CHAPTER
18 Managing Drug Treatment

Drug therapy for rheumatoid arthritis is frequently confusing and frustrating for the patient. It begins with the inability to diagnose rheumatoid arthritis quickly and effectively, which remains difficult even as the twentieth century comes to a close.

Physicians are often criticized because of two complicating, conflicting characteristics. They usually must rely on partial diagnosis because complete quantitative diagnosis is not possible. Then, the course of arthritis is variable with spontaneous remissions often occurring. The only scientific way to overcome these obstacles is to conduct lengthy studies on large numbers of people with rheumatoid arthritis. Such studies require large sums of money, which are not forthcoming. Drug companies study the disease, but the scope of their studies is oriented specifically toward individual drug therapy.

Drugs for arthritis evolved from herbal or other treatments, which has always been a process of trial and error. Indeed, some herbs date to over 3,000 years, with the most universally effective drug being common aspirin, which began as a folk remedy, dried willow bark.

ASPIRIN

Acetylsalicylic acid, common aspirin, is found as salicylates in many plants, especially willow bark. Willow bark as an analgesic is probably as old as man himself. Aspirin was synthesized (made in the laboratory) in 1855 and has been the most widely used drug for arthritis since 1899.

In 1971 Dr. J. R. Vane, a recent Nobel Prize winner for his research on prostaglandins, demonstrated that aspirin reduced the natural production of the prostaglandin I designated as "antagonistic" in Chapter 3. This accounts for the means by which aspirin reduces the pain and inflammation of arthritis. Unfortunately, although it relieves the effects, it does not appear to slow the progress of the disease.

SIDE EFFECTS OF ASPIRIN

Aspirin has unwanted side effects on the gastrointestinal tract. These range from mild heartburn to gastric pain and nausea from even minor doses in some people. Seventy percent of those who use aspirin daily to relieve arthritis inflammation will lose an excess of over 2 milliliters of blood in the stool. The incidence of problems in the stomach and intestine is high. Some experts claim gastric problems can be found in everyone who uses aspirin.

Animal studies have shown that the reasons are probably found in the prostaglandins' protective effect on the stomach and intestinal lining. Apparently, the antagonistic prostaglandins become beneficial when ulcers are involved. Obviously these observations bring to the fore the potential of a dietary approach if it can reduce aspirin or any drug use by even a small percentage.

Other side effects of aspirin include a reduction of the tendency to form internal blood clots. But this does not interfere with the normal blood clotting you would see if, for example, you cut a finger. Indeed, some physicians prescribe aspirin to reduce the tendency for internal clotting in people at risk for heart attack or stroke.

ASPIRIN AND VITAMIN C

Aspirin will suppress the growth of synovial cells cultured in the test tube or, to be scientific, *in vitro*. If vitamin C and aspirin are used together, however, much better results are obtained than either one by itself. In science we call this a "synergistic" result, because it is unexpected. This type of research, although promising, is only helpful because rat cells *in vitro*, even human cells *in vitro*, are not a real person or to be scientifically correct *in situ*.

The obvious next study was to examine vitamin C levels in blood cells of people on aspirin therapy. Indeed, the researchers recognized immediately that the vitamin C levels were low, and they concluded that people on aspirin therapy should also take supplemental vitamin C. The same advice applies to other anti-inflammatory drugs, which are derivatives or analogs of aspirin.

My conclusion from this research is that if you are on aspirin therapy or other nonsteroid anti-inflammatory drugs (e.g., indomethacin), it is appropriate to take additional vitamin C—up to 500 milligrams daily would probably be appropriate.

ALTERNATIVES TO ASPIRIN— NONSTEROIDAL DRUGS

Aspirin is classified as a nonsteroid anti-inflammatory drug, but has been so widely used for centuries, it has special identification; in short, we simply call it "aspirin." Other nonsteroid anti-inflammatory drugs have been developed by drug companies to compete with aspirin and, hopefully, reduce its toxic side effects while being as effective or more effective than aspirin.

At this time there are over thirteen drugs that are in common use, including indomethacin, sulindac, tolmetin, mefenamic acid, flufenamic acid, diclofenac, ibuprofen, naproxen, fenoprofen, phenylbutazone, azapropazon, piroxicam, diflunisal, and others are being tested.

Most experts in the field recognize that all drugs have effects similar to aspirin. And each one appears to have its unique side effects or other actions. All have shown some anti-inflammatory effects in animal studies, but not all have been proven as effective as aspirin in treating rheumatoid arthritis. Therefore it is trial and error between patient, doctor, and drug.

Side effects on the stomach and intestine are apparently reduced with most of these new drugs. But other side effects emerge; most notably on the mental status of older patients. Headaches, dizziness, an inability to concentrate, and confusion frequently signal that a return to traditional aspirin is necessary. A major advantage of these new drugs is that they have longer periods of efficacy and do not need to be taken as often. In summary, they have some advantages over aspirin and some disadvantages, and they all work on the same system. They inhibit the body's production of the antagonistic prostaglandins.

GOLD

In the early 1930s, medical scientists mistakenly thought that tuberculosis and arthritis had the same infectious origins. This is understandable because a type of arthritis often appears in people who have tuberculosis. Because gold compounds were effective against tuberculosis, doctors reasoned, why not arthritis? The results of gold salts on arthritis were formally reported in the medical literature in 1935. They have been used by rheumatologists ever since.

In general, gold is felt to be effective in long-term therapy for people who can tolerate its side effects. One study indicated that it slows the erosive degeneration of the joints over a period of 28 to 36 months. Other studies have shown mixed results but, in general, they indicate some clinical improvement in mobility, grip strength, and a reduction in the amount of analgesic drugs such as aspirin required.

Therefore gold therapy is not curative, but hopefully it will reduce the progress of arthritis development in the long term. In this regard, it appears to be a third line of defense; possibly for some it is the last-ditch effort for people who don't respond to aspirin or other nonsteroidal medication.

SIDE EFFECTS OF GOLD

Every drug has side effects; drugs come into use because the side effects are less severe than the beneficial effects. Gold therapy has side effects that often lead to discontinued use in over 25%, but less than 50% of patients. Therefore the side effects are significant if the "drop-out" rate is high.

Side effects range from mild rash in over 60% of patients to serious kidney problems in about 2.5% of patients. Complications of about 5% can also appear in blood chemistry, which range from mild to very severe. For these reasons, blood and urine chemistry amalyses are necessary precautions that should be taken regularly; indeed, most research physicians recommend this before each administration during the first six months of therapy and regularly, but less frequently, after that.

In general, there are no known interactions with nutrients; therefore this dietary plan should not interfere with gold therapy and vice versa. Indeed, this diet is so nutritionally sound it should be supportive and should reduce both the level and duration of therapy.

Gold accumulates in many of the major organs, including the liver, kidneys, and spleen. Although this is not surprising, it undoubtedly imposes metabolic stress on the body. Thus the maintenance of sound nutritional status is imperative. This diet and its basic supplement plan should be excellent for that purpose.

PENICILLAMINE

Penicillamine decreases the immune complexes in rheumatoid arthritis. It appears similar to gold in efficacy and would be fourth line of defense if gold is third. Clinical results indicate that it appears to reduce swelling, the rheumatoid factor, the number of joints involved, and the subjective pain that develops.

SIDE EFFECTS OF PENICILLAMINE

About 50% of patients who start penicillamine therapy can still continue after one year. It has side effects similar to gold therapy, ranging from mild rash (44% of patients) to serious blood and kidney problems in fewer members. It also appears to induce an autoimmune syndrome in some people. This is a serious concern to any physician and is carefully monitored.

(One side effect is that hypogeusia—a word that means taste perception—is dulled.) Although this usually passes in about three months, it produces a loss in appetite. This is a good reason for people on penicillamine to follow a sound diet and supplement plan.

NUTRITIONAL EFFECTS OF PENICILLAMINE

Penicillamine is a chelating agent that will interfere with metal absorption (e.g., iron). Therefore to prevent iron or other metal deficiency, penicillamine should be taken about 1½ hours after meals. It should not be used at the same time that supplements containing minerals are used. In fact, because supplements should be taken with meals, it would be best to delay the use of penicillamine for 1½ to 2 hours. It might be helpful if your physician agrees to double up on the basic supplement plan.

STEROIDS

Injection of corticosteroids into the arthritic joint often brings remarkable relief. Unfortunately, the relief is not usually sustained, and therefore steroid therapy is useful as support for other forms of therapy.

Corticosteroids affect several systems in the body; they suppress inflammation, which is the major objective of their use. This reduction is brought about by the effects they have on the immune system and their ability to reduce prostaglandin production.

The dramatic relief from steroid use appears to be strictly symptomatic. That means it relieves the symptoms but has no effect on the underlying disease. This relief, however, is so dramatic that there is a tendency to increase the dosage to gain further relief and, as this is done, the side effects begin to become more obvious, and they are not trivial.

Side effects of steroid use range from skin ailments to seizures and many adverse reactions in between. None of them are trivial—like the rash that goes away—so physicians use steroids with great caution.

At present, low-dose oral steroid administration is sometimes used as an adjunct to other drug therapies to relieve symptoms while the drugs are beginning to take effect. Or steroid injection is administered to relieve severe symptoms. But side effects clearly outweigh the beneficial effects, so steroid use should be severely limited.

Nutritional interactions have not been clearly identified. The chronic use of steroids produces so many side effects, however, that the patient must maintain a good nutritional program. Not only should this dietary commitment be maintained, but additional supplements are certainly appropriate.

IMMUNOSUPPRESSIVE DRUGS

Drugs that suppress the immune system should, in principle, be effective against rheumatoid arthritis. Most of the drugs used (e.g., methotrexate) are chemotherapeutic agents effective in reducing malignancies. Put another way, this is the chemotherapy of cancer applied to arthritis.

Although some success has been observed, no drugs have been studied in detail and on large enough numbers to know the extent of their effectiveness. In general, the side effects and toxicities of these powerful agents could be much more serious than simple rheumatoid arthritis itself. These drugs are generally used where all else has failed or is no longer effective. This means that at this time, these drugs are the last-ditch effort!

NUTRITIONAL EFFECTS

Methotrexate is most commonly used and it interferes with one of the B vitamins, folic acid. Therefore for the drug to be effective, supplements should not be used within 8 hours of taking methotrexate. This allows ample time for the drug to be effective and the body to eliminate the excess.

In the use of all these powerful agents, loss of appetite is a common side effect. Therefore care must be taken to follow this dietary commitment and maintain nutritional status by the use of supplements. Doubling of the supplement could be a basis of insuring your basic nutrition.

ORAL CONTRACEPTIVES— PREVENTION

By using oral contraceptives, young women not only avoid unwanted pregnancy, they reduce their chances of getting rheumatoid arthritis. In a study done in Rochester, Minnesota, a reduction was observed in the number of young women who contracted rheumatoid arthritis. Because the same decline was not observed in men of the same age, an astute scientist suspected oral contraceptives. Sure enough, that appeared to be the difference. This has now been confirmed in two subsequent studies in other countries as well.

This observation does not mean that oral contraceptive users will never get arthritis. In fact, about half of them still get it anyway as young women, but there is no evidence as yet that the resistance persists throughout life. But scientists are continuing to study it by follow-up studies in women from middle to old age.

QUACKERY REVISITED: "COPPER SALTS"

Copper salts (ionic copper) inhibit biosynthesis of the antagonistic prostaglandins. This is well established and the metabolic systems involved are well characterized. In fact, they appear to work similarly to gold salts in this respect.

Copper bracelets have been used by arthritics as a form of "folk medicine" for decades—if not centuries. And for decades it has been branded quackery by the government, Arthritis Foundation, health columnists, and me! In short, everyone has jumped on the bandwagon, declaring "Fraud!" All that occurred before research began to uncover the relationship between the antagonistic prostaglandins and inflammation. Indeed, the existence of the other beneficial prostaglandins was even unknown. In fact, some medical scientists now speak of the prostaglandins as though there is only one. Therefore an analytical look at some anecdotal observations is in order.

FOLK MEDICINE—ITS WISDOM

In a previous book, *Making the Vitamin Connection,* I showed how folk wisdom in nutrition had incredible survival value for large populations. Sayings like "an apple a day," "every child needs the January sun," or "fish on Friday," or the addition of a pinch of limestone to tortillas by Mexican mothers to add calcium to the diet, all helped people to thrive when it was difficult to obtain sufficient nourishment. Chauvinistically they were called old wives' tales, which was one way of saying they aren't meaningful. But they are!

Making the Vitamin Connection illustrates that when something survives for years, there's something of value in it. In contrast, many things that don't have value are usually discarded. When something better is identified, they use it; for example, doctors don't use garlic oil to dress wounds in place of more potent antibiotics to prevent infection.

Copper bracelets interact with some people's perspiration to dissolve significant amounts of copper, which penetrates the skin by the process of percutaneous absorption and enters the circulatory system. Although studies comparing copper bracelets with aluminum bracelets suggest that copper does help relieve the inflammation, it clearly warrants further study because there are much more effective means of getting copper ions to the inflammatory site than by the use of a bracelet. But until more research is conducted, copper bracelets cannot do any harm and in spite of the previous branding as "quackery," they might benefit some people.

REFLECTIONS ON DRUG THERAPY

Pharmaceutical science is making great strides in treating arthritis from a scientific, as opposed to strictly an empirical approach. Without doubt, this will bring new and far more effective drug therapy with minimal side effects.

At this time however, I cannot help but be concerned that some of the existing therapy (e.g., gold shots continued for ten years or more) might be worse than the disease itself. But the American approach to illness has traditionally been through medication and the entire system—education through insurance—supports it.

Why authoritative agencies and physicians themselves reject out of hand the possibility that diet can have a significant effect on supporting drug therapy is confusing. In a journal they will report treatment of twenty-seven people with a drug, and if only a few have some success—albeit minor—it will get extensive recognition. In contrast, the notion that diet can help to restore balance to the prostaglandins and optimize drug therapy gets rejected out of hand. But more, the diet can only do good and can do no harm.

Indeed, the side effects of some drugs can be so devastating that in the long term they almost certainly will shorten life and reduce its quality. Therefore if a dietary commitment has any chance of reducing drug dosage or eliminating their use, it should be as welcome as a cool breeze on a hot day.

REDUCING DRUG USE

A physician's objective is to cure his or her patient. In most cases that is exactly what happens, but arthritis is usually different because it is always there; sometimes in remission, sometimes flaring up, depending on many things. So the doctor's objective, by necessity, shifts to keeping it minimized.

Placed in the context of drug therapy, this diet plan will help your body produce a balance between the antagonistic and beneficial prostaglandins. In published clinical studies, this approach has already reduced inflammation and pain, on average, by over 20 to 50% and more in specific cases. Therefore a reduction of drug use should be possible; in specific cases it can be reduced to zero.

The reduction of the medication must be approached by experimentation, however, through collaboration of the patient and the physician. One thing is certain: Only you know how you feel; your doctor must take your word on that. In addition, he or she would like to see you reduce your drug intake as much as possible, and so will be pulling for you as well. Your doctor can precisely evaluate chemical and physical changes, but relies on you to explain how you feel. You should insist on one thing: that he or she be positive. Tell your doctor none of this "diet can't do anything" talk. That's simply sour grapes.

CHAPTER
19 Resisting Quackery

Arthritis and quackery go together like milk and honey. Indeed, whenever a debilitating disease exists, which has no clearly identifiable cure, quackery rushes in to fill the void. Cures, treatments, and nostrums abound.

Arthritis is especially susceptible to quackery because its periods of flare-up are usually unpredictable until you follow this plan, and they usually subside with time. It follows that if some treatment is applied while the flare-up is occurring, both the designer of the treatment and his or her afflicted victim conclude that the treatment works. If the inflammation and its pain subside (go into remission) for a period of weeks, or even months, the purveyor of the treatment has another follower if not a disciple to sell his or her cure. If the attack recurs quickly, the victim usually seeks a different treatment or one that is currently in vogue.

Because arthritis is a joint disease, the treatments often take on some external, physical application such as a "field force" or some other sophisticated-sounding application of electronics. Indeed, history teaches that arthritis treatment is rife with applications. Most of these extend from the simple application of heat to the joint, which brings temporary relief to the joint. This is especially true if the flare-up has been brought on by a change in the weather. But these treatments have no relationship to diet, and I simply want the reader to beware and recognize that they don't work. And if they bring temporary relief, it is probably the result of heat being applied to the aching joint.

Pills, nostrums, and elixers have been sold to arthritics for as long as we know. In fact, the most commonly prescribed drug—aspirin—first appeared as "willow bark," which was and has always been the common cure-all that works. Diet has often been attempted, prescribed, and even scientifically tested. Now we know why some relief was realized through diet.

The simplest diet is to starve oneself, possibly taking only water and fruit juice. It usually worked for arthritics. Today we know it worked because it could have removed the source of sensitivity. And it could have reduced the tendency to produce the antagonistic prostaglandins.

Similar conclusions can be drawn about vegetarian diets, which have prevailed for literally thousands of years. In fact, the vegetarian diet approach has reemerged from time to time and has accumulated a wide following. But this approach has also been branded as quackery without long-term testing. In hindsight, we know it probably helped, but didn't go far enough. The diet in this book goes about as far as we can in using commonly available foods.

There is another level of pills and nostrums that goes beyond diet. These pills purport either to cure or bring relief to arthritics. They consist of ingredients ranging from snake venom to extracts of exotic clams. Snake venom sounds dangerous and clam extract, although probably harmless, could have an offensive odor. But if the use of such materials is not inherently dangerous, it is dangerous because it diverts the sufferer from treatment that can help—and that is quackery.

COMMON SENSE SHOULD PREVAIL

Although I've said it already, I'll say it again: Arthritis is not curable in the sense that appendicitis can be cured, that an infection can be cured or that an illness—like measles—runs its course. Once established, it remains; even if it clears up completely, the potential for recurrence remains.

Therefore any simple device, pill, or nostrum that purports to "cure" should be avoided. At this time they simply don't exist.

PART V

Getting It All Together: People Helping People

CHAPTER
20 Mental Conditioning

A sculptor was asked how he could create such a beautiful statue from a piece of stone. His reply was surprising: "The statue is in the stone; all I do is chip away the residue." The sculptor visualizes the statue, sketches it, then maintains that vision as he carefully eliminates the excess stone.

So it is with life. We've got to visualize what we want to become—visualize ourselves achieving that goal. If the objective is realistic, even if it is a "stretch" for you, it can be achieved. Gaining control over your arthritis is no different than any other objective.

In this chapter I want you to explore how far you are willing to stretch, how you "visualize" yourself, and how you want others to know you.

SUCCESS BEGINS WITH GOALS

When I began working on this diet, I found myself involved with two groups of people: those who wanted to transfer responsibility to others and those who wanted to take responsibility for themselves. More important, I could see the former become the latter if they would only reduce this diet to daily tasks. They learned that success is within themselves if they proceed, one step at a time, toward a realistic, clearly defined goal.

THE BAG STORY

A rather heavy woman approached me at a meeting and asked if this diet would relieve the pain in her knees. Realizing that the diet would definitely help if by nothing else than losing weight, I said, "Only if you will make a commitment to losing ten pounds by following the diet." She immediately replied that she simply couldn't lose weight because diets never worked for her. I told her this diet would if she would give it a chance and monitor her progress with a fat bag. I explained that the fat bag is simply a cloth sack, which she could buy or make. Then, I instructed her to purchase a 10-pound bag of sand or gravel from an aquarium or garden supply store. Each time she lost a pound she should add a pound of sand to the cloth sack, which she should put in a prominent place and carry around from time to time. Within five weeks she had lost 10 pounds and was working on another ten! She bought another bag—the first one was in the family trophy case—full!

The fat bag externalized her daily goal of losing weight and transferred her major objective to a simple task—filling the bag! The arthritis pain diminished from both the weight loss and food changes. She enjoyed newly earned freedom and mobility and an exhilaration she had forgotten since she was a young girl.

Set an objective, reduce it to some daily tasks, and you will succeed!

A SIMPLE SYSTEM THAT WORKS

Objectives work best when we're constantly reminded of them. It follows then that we've got to use the facilities—and people—available to remind us. I have a simple system that works for me; I'll explain it for you.

Write your objectives and goals clearly on 3 × 5 note cards. Keep one set attached to the refrigerator with magnets—in our house the refrigerator is the family bulletin board. Recruit your loved ones, especially your children, to help, and your objectives on one bulletin board will maintain their support. It works!

Carry a set of objective cards with you so you are reminded that we want this plan to become habit. Place one more set on your dresser or wherever you get ready in the morning and evening so you'll see them first thing and last thing each day.

Sound corny?

It's not.

What's corny is the notion that you could have a chronic disease and not use every resource at your disposal to improve the health you've got and reduce the illness to its absolute minimum. In that light, simple note cards are monuments to human willpower and positive mental attitude.

OBJECTIVE SETTING FOR ARTHRITIS

Your broad objective can be simply stated, "Maximize personal control over arthritis." Notice this doesn't include or exclude doctors, diet, medicine, exercise, or anything. It simply states that you want to have as much control over this illness as possible.

This broad objective should be reduced to daily tasks,

which control each variable at your disposal. We have already explored each one—diet, medication, exercise—and when you finish this chapter, you'll have a start on mental outlook.

Diet is the first line of control most of us have over our health. Indeed, when Hippocrates said, in 400 B.C., "let food be thy medicine," he recognized the control it can have over our health. Unfortunately, most people allow that responsibility to be taken by other people—mother, spouse, friends— and it takes willpower to get it back. Set some food-related objectives that are so clear you can't miss. That way you will regain control.

GOAL I
Find Your Flare Points

If you're fortunate enough to have flare-ups due to food, you're a lucky person indeed, because you're in control. Most of the people who follow this diet plan have identified foods that cause their arthritis to flare up. The more systematically they approach their quest, the more successful they are. I know you've heard it before, but you've got to keep the food diary. If you eat the wrong thing, your joints usually respond within 12 hours.

Goal I: Keep a food diary and find your flare foods. Once found, you're in control.

GOAL II
Make This Diet Become Habit

"One Bite at a Time"—

While we've talked about diet all through this book, you must still put it into effect "one bite at a time." Reducing it to a daily menu is all that's required. And depending on your circumstances, it means planning one food day at a time.

You're the controller and must use your resources effectively. The best way is to plan each day the evening before. In this way you will do two things automatically: Plan your food and food supplements, and start taking control of your time.

Use your food diary to write down what you plan to do the next day. At the end of that day you can simply write a report card on how you did—and how you feel—then what you're going to do the next day.

Let me give you an analogy.

My family sails. We take our 47-foot ketch, *La Scala*, out on day sails in San Francisco Bay, and also on the Pacific Ocean for trips of several days. At the end of each day I write into the log a narrative of what, when, who, why, and observations of what we learned and what I plan to do the next day. It's amazing how useful it is to look back when we're in a new situation to see what we learned in similar situations.

It doesn't seem corny to keep a log in the context of going to sea on the West Coast, which is terribly unforgiving of mistakes. In fact, the sea is completely indifferent to the frailties of the boat or the crew. I have never met anyone who thinks my log is corny; in fact, most skippers who see it start one of their own.

You're a skipper—start one now!

GOAL III
Weight Control

Use a Fat Bag

Give yourself the test in Chapter 13 to get your weight under control. If you're not overweight, think exercise to firm up; then read on because you're going to start helping others and you'll need some preparation.

After you take the test, climb on a scale and note your weight. Then get started with a fat bag and write down your weight goal clearly. It can be in pounds, it can be in inches, but use a fat bag to monitor progress. By using the food diary, willpower, and the fat bag, you'll reach your goal. If you're a typical American, you'll want to go further and lose more; but remember, one pound at a time.

People who set out to lose a lot of weight (e.g., 150 pounds) often fail. They fail because weight can only come off consistently at about 1½ or 2 pounds each week. At that rate it could take years to lose 100 pounds, seemingly forever. But, in 10-pound increments it's only about five or six weeks and, with a fat bag, you can hold progress in your hand. Your trophy case will have ten trophies!

I've met lots of people who have lost more than 100 pounds in 10-pound increments and they get a new lease on life in exchange for their perseverence.

GOAL IV
Stress Control

Mental Conditioning

I'm often asked, "What should I take to control stress?" and I can detect the stress in the voice even if it's over a telephone. My heart goes out to the person at the other end because I want to give a simple answer and I can't. Controlling stress requires conditioning for stress. The next question I get is how do you condition for stress?

Conditioning for stress is no different than the way in which athletes train for an event. The practice for stress is mental as compared with physical practice for an athletic objective.

POSITIVE THINKING

Mental conditioning can be practiced all day every day. This is in contrast to physical conditioning, which requires special equipment, time, and other restrictions. Mental conditioning requires much more self-discipline, however. Positive thinking, positive mental attitude, positive recognition, and positive action without reward are necessary. Let's explore how each of these helps.

In each situation you must first apply the maxim that something positive exists in every situation. Find the positive and build on it; don't dwell on the negative. One woman spoke to me once with a beautiful example; the conversation went like this:

"Dr. Scala, I've got a flare-up like I haven't had in months."

I immediately started to console her. "No," she immediately responded. "I'm glad; you see, we went to a party last night and since being on your diet, I haven't had chopped liver." I nodded in agreement as she continued. "This flare-up proves a point; I know that I shouldn't eat chopped liver and drink so much wine."

That is an excellent example of positive thinking; she saw a positive in what other people would have seen as a negative. Find the positive in every situation and build on it. Positive thinking will become automatic and as much a habit as this way of eating.

Another example: I had chipped a tooth. Shortly after a colleague, Nancy, came into my office. I told her of the chipped tooth. Her reply was immediate. "Oh, Jim, think of it, you'll be able to see Dr. Giers," and she beamed a big grin. She went on, "He's always so enjoyable to talk with and he'll have that tooth like new."

The ability to see positive in a chipped tooth is truly positive thinking. She is about the best example I know of a person whose thought process automatically responds to everything in a positive manner. But it's the result of positive self-discipline all her life. With Nancy a positive outlook is automatic.

POSITIVE MENTAL ATTITUDE

A positive mental attitude is a little more subtle. It requires searching for the silver lining in the cloud that's on the horizon. It is an attitude that the future is always a little brighter than the present. It's the attitude that allows people to see beyond the years and build for a brighter future.

The Roman philosopher, Cicero, wrote of people planting

olive orchards, recognizing that they would derive little benefit from them in their lifetime. He observed that they would
be there to feed future generations. That is a positive mental
attitude—to constantly strive for a better future.

A second excellent example is my mother. I found a bag of
dried peach pits in her study. When I offered to throw them
out, her reply was immediate: "Oh no, Jimmy, I often substitute for the fourth grade and I use them to have the children
make turkeys." She went on to explain how she uses tooth-
picks, glue, cotton, and some paper to make miniature turkeys with third- and fourth-grade students around Thanksgiving.
You think, so what? Well, at the time my mother was 76
years old! She was still planning how she would keep students
productively occupied as a substitute teacher. That fall she
was often asked to substitute and she used those peach pits!
And now, at age 80, she still does the same thing. It's called
positive mental attitude.

POSITIVE RECOGNITION

Positive recognition is the easiest of all. You only have to
say something nice to someone. Suppose it's a waitress. Before
you order say, "What a nice smile you've got," or "That color
is very becoming," or "Your walk sure has a bounce to it."
The idea is simple: Find some way to recognize something
good in your fellow humans. This recognition will come back
to you many times over; you'll start to find good things in
yourself. If you learn to find and call attention to something
good in others, it will become second nature to you and
fertilize your growing positive thoughts and attitude.

POSITIVE ACTION

Last is action. You need to love yourself, and there's no better way than doing something positive anonymously. Help a stranger, give an anonymous gift, send a note to someone and sign it, "an admirer." But, also do it so people know you do it. If someone does something well, give them a "thumbs up" sign. A "thumbs up" is easy. It's a short note from you to them with something positive for them; such as: Dear Kim, I sure enjoyed the way you played that piece on the piano yesterday. It showed excellent progress on your part. Love, Dad. To an employee, to a friend, to a boss, a colleague—to anyone.

Sound corny? Don't kid yourself; think of how you'd feel if you got one! If you start now, you'll be surprised how effectively these actions will condition your positive mental processes. You'll need it because you've got an illness that won't quit; stress that won't quit. The only way to beat stress is to maintain mental conditioning as much as a world-class athlete maintains physical conditioning.

ONE LAST TIME: MENTAL ATTITUDE

You Are What You Eat

Mental attitude is everything; indeed, I call it human spirit. It can turn a seemingly hopeless situation into one that becomes the starting point for greatness. It all begins with nourishment—both mental and physical.

In this chapter I've tried to make you aware of some concepts of mental health, to give you some "food for thought." It's all homage to the concept of you're the one who controls what goes into your body: your destiny.

Just as this book is about improving life through diet, so is it about mental nourishment. As you apply these dietary concepts so are you applying a mental recognition.

You are unique. There is no living thing precisely like you in this universe, and the nourishment you put into your body is your public statement of the importance you place on that uniqueness; the dignity you place on your body. To improve your health you must improve your physical nourishment and your spiritual nourishment. That is the food you feed your body and the food you feed your mind.

CHAPTER
21 Shoulders to Lean On: Support Groups

People need people. This phrase has more meaning for arthritis than any other chronic illness, excepting possibly alcoholism. Alcoholism is a chronic illness with hereditary aspects like arthritis. Alcoholism can be controlled but not cured, just like arthritis. The entire foundation of Alcoholics Anonymous is that you must control your illness yourself and you need the support of others, If I make them sound similar, it's because they are! Everyone accepts self-help groups for alcoholism; why not arthritis?

My comparison to Alcoholics Anonymous is dramatic; I hope it got your attention. Now explore how arthritics can help arthritics.

By now you know that there are about 100 illnesses that can be classified as some form of arthritis. Each one has its own characteristics and affects each person differently. Further, new methods of treatment are constantly emerging, new clothing, new concepts such as this dietary plan. The things people can learn about arthritis from each other are too numerous to count.

I asked one woman what was the most memorable thing she learned at her arthritis discussion group. It was the side effects of the penicillamine therapy her physician was using.

He had mentioned the side effects in passing, but she didn't hear him for any number of reasons, probably the pressure of time. But she mentioned how she felt at the arthritis group and another woman told her what to expect, how long it would last, and helped her learn to cope. But there's much more to derive from groups than just helpful hints.

Possibly the most helpful outcome is indirect. It feeds the positive thinking we just explored. You will see how other people cope—or don't cope. You will realize that no matter how difficult things may seem, there are other people who have it worse, and you can thank God that you have the health you do. Most important if you go to an arthritis help group, you should go to accomplish two things: learn from others and help others.

If you take this dietary commitment seriously, you will have a common bond of discussion—a point from which to help others and from which to learn from others. You will learn much from others by listening to what causes flare-ups in them and how they eat to avoid inflammation. I could never begin to include all the foods that fit into this dietary plan; it would take volumes. Nor could I even identify all the variations that make the foods interesting and palatable. Obviously, if you start a group just to discuss dietary issues, there is no end to the meetings and discussions you can have. But, there's more.

MEDICAL KNOWLEDGE

The Arthritis Foundation publishes excellent literature on arthritis. And, although they don't give dietary considerations fair treatment, the literature they prepare provides an endless basis for discussion. Indeed, they have chapters in many areas and will be happy to serve as the catalyst for discussion.

Physicians who specialize in arthritis—and no matter where you live, there's one in your area—are flattered by invitations to speak. They can explain the methods of medication, the side effects, why one course of therapy is chosen over another. They can learn from you—yes, they will never know your illness like you do—and the subtleties of what causes flare-ups will help them with other patients. No matter what you've been told, communication is a two-way street with physicians.

I have spoken with arthritis discussion groups and have learned more from them than they from me. Sure, I tell them all about prostaglandins, EPA and diet. I discuss the history of arthritis and other interesting things. I learn much about them from their questions. I learn how they cope and how theory gets put into practice. As Confucius said, "To teach is to learn," and a good teacher always learns more than his students.

HELP OTHERS

The most important benefit from an arthritis support group is what you can do for others. I have the advantage of speaking all over the world and I meet people everywhere. None are as desperate or scared as young women who have just learned they have arthritis. No combat veteran, no witness to terror, no survivor of tragedy can have a more frightened look in their eyes. You can do so much to make these people learn that they can cope, they can help their physician gain control, they can lead a productive life, raise a family, laugh, and have fun. You can set an example with your own positive thinking, your optimistic outlook, and your support. You can send them a "thumbs up."

But, the group does more. There are times when the inflammation and the pain reduce the outlook to an all-time low. These are the times when people want to quit. And that's when they need maximum support; they need someone to carry them with mental support, to visualize the sunshine over a dark horizon.

PERIPHERAL SUPPORT SPEAKERS

This plan emphasizes diet, so dieticians would make excellent invited speakers for any support group. They also make excellent counselors. But don't stop there. Invite exercise physiologists, therapists, chiropractors who work with arthritics, and others. Further, they should be able to discuss the benefits of various types and levels of exercise for differing levels of severity.

Dieticians who take this dietary commitment seriously can speak and help design menus and foods that meet all the criteria. But don't invite dieticians who are too mentally constipated to look beyond the basic food groups and recognize the need for basic supplementation. These are fundamental to your new way of life.

Nurses who work with rheumatologists are informative speakers. Nurses are the unsung heroes of modern medicine. They usually have more time to observe subtleties of arthritis than the physician. Their ability and willingness to explain self help is endless. A little recognition of them will go a long way.

Clothing specialists who make garments that help ease sensitivity should also be invited. These people can learn much from you that will accrue to their economic advantage. So, once more your efforts will reach others.

Pharmacists can talk about the medications that are most frequently used—and abused, those that are most current. More important, the pharmacist can alert you to drug interactions.

IT'S THE PEOPLE

No person is alone; we must help our fellows—our shipmates. That's why we must seek out people who can teach us and who we can teach. I have never met a person who was too old to learn or was too old to teach. Nor have I ever met a person who cannot derive mental nourishment from helping another person. When people communicate about a common cause, synergy emerges that lifts the spirits like a phoenix to heaven. That is why people are so important.

CHAPTER
22 Real Success Stories

I want you to see yourself in the pages of this chapter. In the development of this plan I have corresponded with many people. Indeed, I have spoken often with many of them, gotten to know them personally. From these discussions several characteristics about arthritis emerged that helped me to understand the illness and the people.

I realized that there is a pattern of its emergence as an illness. In my opinion, after many discussions, stress is inexorably involved in arthritis. Similarly, mental attitude is involved.

The medical approach is unclear. Drugs such as aspirin and its more modern counterparts help a great deal. But with gold shots I'm confused; a question arises: Should the cure continue for ten years, and after so long is it worse than the illness?

Diet is undoubtedly effective in helping to relieve the inflammation. But there's more. Specific foods clearly cause flare-ups in some people but not others. If it is an allergy, it is not in the classic sense.

Weight loss in overweight people helps in two ways. It obviously removes a serious stress on joints, but it also gives a renewed self-image. And self-image, like positive thinking, can move mountains.

Exercise emerges as an elixer that cannot be discounted. And, even the most restricted people find the means to exercise, and it's helpful.

I hope you will enjoy these lessons from personal experience as much as I have.

For obvious reasons I have not used peoples' correct names in these pages. They were kind enough to share their experiences with me so that others may benefit, and I respect their anonymity.

STRESS—THE STARTING POINT

Adults who get arthritis can usually trace its beginnings to some specific event. Most common is childbirth, but there are many others. From my own personal observations, I have concluded that stress of some kind is always involved.

Linda's Story—Childbirth

Linda has three children and has been taking weekly gold injections for five years. She is finding the dietary commitment helpful.

Dear Dr. Scala:

My arthritis just appeared after I had my first baby. At first the doctor wasn't sure but he took some tests and told me. My knees had swollen and my wrists hurt at first.

While I was carrying my other two children I felt wonderful. There wasn't a hint of the problem. I never ached or even felt stiff.

After my second child I was so bad that I had to stay in the hospital a week. Everything ached and I felt terrible.

Linda went on to tell me that she wished she could be pregnant all the time without having children. As she put it, when she was pregnant she felt great. After her third child her arthritis progressively worsened.

Betty's Story—An Accident

Betty has written to me often. She is faithful to this plan, and the benefits she has derived are gratifying. The way in which her arthritis appeared is typical:

> I had to drop a cake off at church and I left my car without putting the brake on. It started rolling so I put the cake down and ran to stop it I slipped on the ice and was pinned between my car and another car. My right knee was very badly bruised.
>
> I spent a week in the hospital and then a week at home before I could go back to work. At the end of the week in the hospital my wrist started hurting. While at home it continued to bother me and became swollen so I asked the doctor to look at it. He thought it was from work, the way I opened and wrapped packages. At the end of my first week at home, the week after the accident, my ankle started hurting and it was swollen. It got red and sore.

With the sore ankle and the wrist hurting, her doctor tested for arthritis. Sure enough, Betty tested positive for arthritis. Betty could always control the inflammation and pain with standard oral medication. However, it progressed to the point where she couldn't continue to work.

Nancy's Story—An Accident

Nancy has arthritis in her right leg, right shoulder, right elbow, wrist, middle and index fingers of the right hand. It started about twenty-five years previous in an auto accident in which she was injured on her right side. After she left the hospital she noticed that when she woke up, the middle finger of her right hand would ache—a dull ache, not sharp pain. It progressed to her wrist, elbow and shoulder. Now it's in her spine and right leg. She relates that it took about two years to spread.

Nancy has used alfalfa and this diet to rid herself of arthritis. She sticks to the diet and takes medication only when necessary.

Leslie's Story—Stress of Divorce

Leslie is about 30 years old. She's had five children and was in excellent health. Then her marriage failed through no fault of her own; her husband sought and received a divorce.

Right after the divorce she noticed that she would wake up with pain in both hands and shoulders. When the pain was accompanied by swelling (about four months later), she went to the doctor.

Leslie's doctor did all the standard tests and the diagnosis was positive. She had progressed from aspirin (which made her nauseated) to clinoril. Then she was given oral gold and cortisone.

Leslie has regressed to a poor condition; it has affected her hands, toes, shoulders, and knees. Her muscles are bad and now her jaw has become involved.

As evidence of the continuing stress, she is unable to sleep and is so tired she cannot get up in the morning. This stress spiral, I have come to believe, is typical of arthritis—it feeds on itself. The illness is so devastating that it creates fear of what is happening, the future looks bleak, the medication makes you miserable, and the stress gets worse. As the stress progresses so does the medication. It is a vicious spiral.

Beth's Story—The Affair

Beth developed arthritis following the stress of a serious marital problem. Her arthritis coincided with her extramarital affair. She met an old flame while visiting with her mother.

One thing led to another—call it biology—and the effect of a rigid Catholic upbringing. Guilt can be a terrible stress on the body and cause anyone to become run down. In Beth's case, the exhilaration of finding herself still desirable was finally overcome by the guilt and close destruction of her marriage. It was devastating! But all is fine now; her marriage is sound, and she has the arthritis under control.

In contrast to Leslie, Beth either took control and stopped the stress or, for other reasons, the progression of the arthritis stopped. She got along on aspirin (or a little stronger medication) until she started the diet. Now she's off everything!

Men have usually traced their arthritis to some sports injury. Very often it's a knee that was injured in baseball or football. But often the arthritis starts later in life, and with some type of stress—usually in the form of illness.

Ruth's Story—Willpower

Ruth had arthritis for several years and finally realized that the spiral of anxiety, depression, and sleeplessness was destroying her. She decided that was all she would tolerate. She said that from that day on it has not gotten any worse and with this diet and her doctor's help, she is getting better. She sleeps well, eats well, and exercises regularly.

Connie's Story—It Just Came

Connie woke up one morning at 16 years of age and just felt terrible; she couldn't get up, she couldn't walk. The arthritis traveled from her knees to her hands and wrists. Wrist rotation froze within a month. The next step was gold shots—and they helped. In her own words, "I could tell when it was time for the shots because I hurt so."

Connie and I could find no stress other than normal high school activities. About one year before the onset of arthritis, however, she was so tired she would go to sleep as soon as she arrived home from school until the next morning, with a short break for dinner. This went on for weeks; her doctor tested for mononucleosis and a thyroid problem. Neither test was positive and she eventually came out of it.

In hindsight, the fatigue should have been pursued further because she had always been such an active person. Such a dramatic change in activity was surely symptomatic of an illness.

STRESS—SOME CONCLUSIONS

Without attempting to practice medicine or to diagnose, I can draw some conclusions. It appears to me that stress is a type of trigger for arthritis. Most women I spoke to could trace the beginnings to a stressful event. And the stress could be either physical or emotional; usually it was some of both.

Working with athletes makes me respect mental over physical power. I now believe that it can go both ways. Guilt and other forms of emotional stress can so drain the body's reserves that a disease can start. And if the researchers who trace arthritis to a virus are correct, emotional stress can reduce the immune capacity enough to let it get started.

Injury obviously does the same thing, but it's more obvious. All the body's reserves are challenged and occasionally the arthritis wins.

Childbirth often has a prominent role as the starting point. While the woman is pregnant, arthritis is often dormant; obviously the hormonal influence on the immune system is at work. It probably explains why women who use the birth control pill are less likely to have arthritis, following pregnancy.

FOOD DIARY RESULTS

Sensitivities

On a recent TV talk show a physician showed film clips to illustrate how food sensitivities aggravated arthritis. The physician injected an extract of certain foods into selected patients. The results were dramatic. Within hours, joints would swell, become immobile; pain was obvious in the expression of the volunteer's face. The doctor made his point in vivid living color.

Unfortunately—or fortunately—most sensitivities are not that clear. Moreover, most of us can't afford to have food extracts prepared and tested by taking capsules containing them or having injections. But experience with the personal discoveries people have made using food diaries illustrates that it is not as clear and well defined as the doctor so dramatically illustrated.

Elizabeth's Story—Milk and Eggs

Elizabeth faithfully keeps a food diary. It didn't take long to discover that dairy products—milk, yogurt, most cheese—will bring on swelling, pain, and reduced mobility of her knees, ankles, and wrists. But her experience with eggs is interesting.

"If I eat two eggs three days running, on the third day I can feel it coming. By the fourth day I can hardly get out of bed." Elizabeth can use eggs, however. "I ate a poached egg once when my niece stayed with me, and felt fine. With a little experimenting I learned that I can tolerate an egg now and then. It's only when I have more than one at a time, or one each day."

Elizabeth clearly asked the salient question: "Dr. Scala, can that be correct, could I tolerate one egg from time to time? Or could it all be in my head?"

I told her it isn't in her head; after all, she carefully evaluated her response to certain foods. She got in touch with her body and knows its limits. Whatever it is in eggs that causes the flare-up simply must not exceed her threshold level.

Alice's Story—Tomatoes

Alice and her husband live in the Midwest. The diet worked very well for her. In her own words, an excerpt: "I feel so much better with my arthritis I can hardly believe it. I have always heard you are what you eat. Now I believe it; thanks to you and my daughter for taking the time to send me your diet."

Alice kept a food diary and by trial and flare-up learned that she cannot eat tomatoes. She can, however, eat potatoes and eggplant. She confirms my notion that the nightshade plants should not categorically be eliminated. Because Alice stays closely with the plan and uses the food diary, she has not identified any other foods that caused trouble.

Patricia's Discovery—Mocha Mix

Patricia cannot use dairy products, even skim milk. She found that it produces inflammation. However, in her own words; "I agree on the advantages of oatmeal. One way to enjoy it for breakfast is to use an artificial 'nondairy' creamer, such as Mocha Mix, Rich, or any vegetable creamer available in the dairy section."

Bernette's Story

Bernette has followed the diet faithfully. She cannot eat grapefruit and tomatoes; in her own words:

"I found I was not able to eat grapefruit as my knees and elbows became sore. Last summer when our tomatoes were producing, I foolishly ate a lot and my joints became very sore, and when I stopped eating tomatoes, the pain and swelling went away. I found since following your diet that my ankles are not puffy at night as they have been for a long time."

Her letter goes on to discuss other things, but it's quite clear that she reacts to certain foods. Most interesting, none of them fall into a pattern—grapefruit and tomatoes are quite different. The disappearance of ankle puffiness is similar to what other people, including physicians, observe.

LOSING WEIGHT

Sometimes I feel that I've found the ideal weight loss diet. Everyone who started the diet did so for arthritis, but every letter or telephone conversation includes a statement about losing weight.

Barb's Story

Barb is a registered nurse who started some friends on the diet. She used two of them as examples to get other people to her arthritis support group. She gives two testimonials in her notice.

Phyllis' story—as told by Barb—goes on to tell how well she feels, reduced pain, and so on; then after four weeks, "There is less cloudiness in her eyes; happily she has lost five pounds."

Frances's story—as told by Barb—explains how well she is doing; for example, in less than a week she felt improvement in her knees, but the weight came at the end—"Frances also is losing unwanted pounds at a rate of 2 pounds a week and who wouldn't feel good about that."

Joyce explains the benefits of the diet and goes on to say, "I have lost ten plus pounds."

Rusty's Story

Let Rusty tell it in her own words: "Since beginning the arthritis diet, my weight has gone from 165 pounds to 145 pounds. That's okay as I'm 5'9" tall and never was heavy until arthritis limited my activity. I've also taken 3 to 4 inches off my waist! That's terrific!!"

Obviously, the diet works effectively as a weight loss diet and, as Rusty put it so clearly, it helps to shift the weight because measurements, not pounds, are what counts. Rusty has a form of osteoarthritis called ankylosing spondylytis and has found much relief from this diet.

EXERCISE

Most people try to exercise and it becomes very difficult as the arthritis gets worse. But one woman, Thelma, described something so beautiful that I feel it should be shared.

Thelma: "I go to the municipal indoor pool and exercise." I quizzed her further: "Do they have a program there?" She replied, "Oh, heavens no, I get into the water and do the exercises you told me to do. In the water it doesn't hurt; I guess it keeps the weight off my knees." I was surprised so I asked if she does it alone. "Oh no, I have lots of friends now and we all do it. Oh some of them have to get in up to their neck because they aren't as good as me, but they are seeing results."

I can't tell you how gratifying it is to see people helping people like that. And the common sense that led them to do it is astounding. So I asked Thelma if it helped. "Well, look at it this way. I used to get a ride to the pool because I couldn't walk that far, and now I walk both ways."

GENERAL RESULTS

Many people have now pursued this diet, and I'll share some short comments in addition to those I've expressed for specific reasons.

Lydia: "I feel I am doing something right now; the signs of arthritis have disappeared."

Elsie: "I am on your arthritis program and have improved quite a lot."

Donna: "I am feeling so much better I should have written sooner."

Alice: "I feel so much better I can hardly believe it."

Elmer (age 81): "I started it April 9th and haven't seen any improvement. I'll stick with it for three more weeks." In three weeks I spoke to Elmer. "I'm starting to see results; I notice I can get right up in the morning now."

Carole (age 31): "I can't tell you how great it feels to be normal again. I am just astonished (she goes on to explain what she can't eat). I don't have a tinge of pain, no soreness. I feel great."

Ursula (reporting on her mother): "We are afraid to be overly optimistic, but she had almost immediate results. As of today her leg and foot are normal, all swelling gone. Her hands look normal; the swelling is gone."

Yvette: "I've been following your diet for a month now and I've noticed a big difference. I'm not as stiff and I have more strength. I feel very good, I have dreams of walking without any more problems."

Joyce: "I felt good to begin with so I don't feel better. I have found that when I have any forbidden foods I experience a flare-up, usually within eight hours or less—most often in my wrists or hands. I do believe that by following this diet the quality of life for many people would improve."

Connie: "I feel great because now I'm doing something positive and the diet works. My doctor will work with me to spread out the gold shots. I've been on them for ten years and would like to reduce them."

CONCLUSIONS

I could go on and on with testimonials. They indicate to me that people gain improvement in their lives and more freedom from the flare-ups that seem so common. If people will only use a food diary and start with the Do's and Don'ts, the quality of their lives will improve.

It has confirmed one very important teaching for me. We are personally responsible for the food we choose and cannot escape the observation that "we are what we eat."

CHAPTER

23 Arthritis and Human Development

Many variations of arthritis exist; they have similarities and differences. Some experts say 100 variations exist. To make it more complex, people can have more than one type at a time; therefore the permutations and combinations are almost endless.

All forms of arthritis are similar in one respect. They have flare-ups and periods of remission. Flare-ups are periods during which they are active—joints are inflamed, pain is apparent. Flare-ups can last from hours or days to months and years. Remissions, in contrast, are periods of dormancy when for all practical purposes the disease doesn't exist. Remissions similarly vary in length.

My curiosity led me to question the historical aspects of arthritis. Is arthritis a disease of modern times or has it always existed in one form or another? Does the future look bright or bleak? Will it be eliminated someday?

200 MILLION YEARS OF OSTEOARTHRITIS

The University of Kansas Natural History Museum has on display the skeleton of an extinct swimming reptile, the platycarpus. It inhabited the shallow sea, which is now the great Midwest, 200 million years ago. All the joints of the left hind limb of this Kansan specimen were deformed by osteoarthritis, and the deformations are similar to those a physician would see in human osteoarthritis today.

Although its animal hosts have changed, osteoarthritis has not changed in over 200 million years. In the Kansan platycarpus, the joints are deformed by bony overgrowths and the joint bones contain increased vascular spaces, just like a physician would see today. One affliction has never changed.

HUMAN HISTORY OF OSTEOARTHRITIS

Our most remote ancestors first roamed the Olduvai Gorge in Africa three million years ago and, one million years later, they lived long enough to get osteoarthritis. One million years ago Java man and 500,000 years ago Lansing man both got osteoarthritis even though they lived in widely separated times and parts of the world. In fact, one specimen of Java man would have been a candidate for a hip replacement if he lived today.

Archaeologists mistakenly named osteoarthritis "cave gout" because it was so common in skeletons of the cave man. It was found in the 40,000-year-old skeletons of Neanderthal man, 7,000-year-old mummies from Egypt and Peru, and 3,000-year-old skeletons from the Indian subcontinent.

Here in the United States excavations of the Mound Builder

Indians from Port Clinton, Ohio, around 850 A.D. indicate that most of the adults had some form of osteoarthritis. Burial sites in other areas, ranging from the Southeast in Alabama to the Southwest in New Mexico and north to Alaska, show quite clearly that native Americans got osteoarthritis—it didn't come over with the pilgrims.

Excavations in England prove the pilgrims weren't spared. Not only did the Roman invaders have osteoarthritis, but so did the Saxons whom they invaded. This isn't meant to be overwhelming; it only shows that osteoarthritis has always been part of the human condition.

In fact, we all get osteoarthritis to some degree. About 97% of people over 65 years old will have some x-ray evidence of osteoarthritis, and 50% will have evidence that is significant. Unlike rheumatoid arthritis and gout, it is not a metabolic or systemic disease; that is, if it occurs in one joint, it does not necessarily spread to others. A hereditary tendency apparently exists, and people who get the disease in one joint early in life often develop it in other joints as they age. This is because the cartilage covering the joint bones is hereditarily weak in all joints and more susceptible to damage than average.

Osteoarthritis is the price we pay for living under the influence of gravity. It is simply the wear and tear on the joints, and it can start with an athletic injury, a common household injury, or "just plain living" from day to day.

RHEUMATOID ARTHRITIS

Unlike osteoarthritis, rheumatoid arthritis is a disease of the soft tissue and doesn't leave a fossil record. Medical archaeologists must search for its evidence among bodies that have been preserved. Consequently, the oldest example of what could pass for rheumatoid arthritis is seen in the 4,700-year-old mummified remains of a Syrian emigrant to

Egypt. When this man lived, he suffered with swollen, deformed joints in his hands, knees, and feet. This, and a few other mummified specimens indicate that rheumatoid arthritis has probably been part of the human condition for about 5,000 years.

However, the absence of rheumatoid arthritis in the Old Testament is puzzling. Because it has such clear characteristic deformities, one would expect it to appear had it been widespread. Therefore it is most noticeable by its absence.

Probably the earliest written description of rheumatoid arthritis appears in ancient Indian literature from about 1000 B.C. Caraka, a physician of that time, identified and described rheumatoid arthritis as a metabolic disorder, which generally involved the joints of fingers, hands, and feet and could spread to all joints. He went even further to describe the involvement of other organs such as the liver, spleen, lungs, and heart.

Caraka's most important contribution was his identification of gum-guggulu (*commiphora mukul*), a plant derivative that is similar in efficacy to some modern anti-inflammatory medications. He also advised heat to help relieve the pain that comes with inflammation, and he recommended that the sufferer be placed in a pile of fermenting barley. (Fermenting barley would be about the correct temperature for pain relief.) He also identified various poultices that create the same mild irritation modern liniments and rubs do today and subsequent heat as prescriptions for relief. They probably were just as effective as today's liniments and rubs.

Six hundred years later in Greece, circa 400 B.C., Hippocrates identified and described two diseases—podagra, which we know as gout, and rheumatoid arthritis. Similarities exist between gout and rheumatoid arthritis, and people can have both together—a fact that created confusion then and still does today. (I will cover gout separately.) Hippocrates had clearly seen the difference between gout and rheumatoid arthritis.

Hippocrates is generally credited with recommending the

chewing of willow bark as a means of relieving pain and inflammation. Although willow bark is an effective source of aspirin (Chapter 18), it was probably widely used before Hippocrates.

Hippocrates described arthritis as a disease that generally appeared in men about age 35. He identified it as beginning in the feet and moving to the hands, where the fingers became slender and cold, whereas the joints became distorted, enlarged, and progressively difficult to use.

At the beginning of the Christian era in 2 A.D., Soranus of Ephesus, a descendant and follower of the school of Hippocrates, described rheumatoid arthritis as a chronic metabolic disease. Although Hippocrates had described it as a disease of men, Soranus observed that it occasionally occurred in women, especially following childbirth. He noted that children seldom contracted it and even eunuchs developed the disease. Because eunuchs didn't get gout, this was a very important distinction.

Soranus left no doubt about rheumatoid arthritis as he accurately described twisted, immovable fingers—often turned sideways—and early morning stiffness. He described the nature of flare-ups, relating them to food, and observed that arthritics could predict the weather. Soranus left little to be said that we don't observe today. But, he left us with a mystery.

Soranus, as Hippocrates before him had done, described arthritis as a disease of men in their thirties. He recognized that it occurred only occasionally in women and seldom in children. This does not square with the statistics of what exists today, and raises two questions. Was the world so chauvinistic at the time that illness in women didn't count? I doubt it! Or did the disease change? I think so!

The next significant descriptions of rheumatoid arthritis came from Thomas Sydenham, an Englishman, in his extensive treatise of 1676—a full, 1,674 years after Soranus! Indeed, that is a long gap, considering the disease has such severity and consequences. If it was only 20% as widespread as it is today, it couldn't have gone unnoticed for so long. We would have expected to see it in art and sculpture as well as the writings of such authors as William Shakespeare.

Sydenham leaves no doubt in his descriptions under the title of Rheumatism that rheumatoid arthritis existed, for he vividly described the inflammation, pain, deformities, and suffering. His descriptions are so accurate they would stand today if placed in modern English.

WHY THE 1,674-YEAR GAP?

The first thought is that life expectancy was so short on average until the 1600s that people didn't survive long enough to get the disease. This is simply not so. People often survived longer than age 40, and the Greek school made it clear that women and children did get the disease. Therefore life expectancy does not account for the gap.

Some medical scientists speculate that the ancient writings and historical evidence don't deal with rheumatoid arthritis as it exists today. In fact, they speculate that what was observed was a complication of gout and osteoarthritis. In fact, they argue that because it doesn't appear in writing and art much before the seventeenth century, that it either got its start or gained new virulence at that time. Indeed, they argue that its absence in the bible, in art, and the early confusion with gout coupled with our modern preoccupation with the disease, caused us to see something in early writings that didn't exist or was no more than a curiosity—a rare occurrence. Clearly, the mummified remains could be a special case of gout with osteoarthritis. They go on to speculate that rheumatoid arthritis evolved from a special form of spondylitis and, consequently, it is a disease of the modern era.

RHEUMATOID ARTHRITIS: SOME SPECULATION

The writings of Caraka in 1000 B.C., the descriptions of Hippocrates in 400 B.C., perpetuated by Soranus in 2 A.D. leave little doubt in my mind that a form of rheumatoid arthritis existed long before the modern era. It was not as widespread nor prevalent, however, and possibly even became dormant. Further, if we use the Eskimos as examples, diet can mitigate against it, which would make it much less noticed.

With increasing population, changes in dietary habits, and poor sanitation, a new more virulent form could have developed. This matches the writings of Caraka and Hippocrates, who place it as a disease of men in contrast to modern epidemiology, which places the burden on women by three to one. In support of those who teach that it evolved from spondylitis, we know that men get spondylitis ten to one.

RHEUMATOID ARTHRITIS: 1850 TO PRESENT

In 1857, the first illustrated account of rheumatoid arthritis appeared. Between 1857 and the early twentieth century, however, a debate continued between physicians who insisted that it was a variation of gout, and others who correctly identified it as a disease in its own right.

The advent of x-ray in 1900 permitted physicians to differentiate between osteoarthritis and rheumatoid arthritis. By 1948, tests were made that identified the factor in blood on which modern diagnosis rests. This "rheumatoid factor" is the dominant diagnostic factor today. It is coupled with other blood, tissue, and x-ray analyses.

We also know today that there is a hereditary predisposition to the disease. This doesn't mean that if one of your parents or grandparents had the disease, you will get it. Indeed, it only means that you are more susceptible to it. If, as modern hypothesis teaches, it is caused by a virus, then the hereditary tendency is more obvious. It is more obvious because of selective sensitivities, selective immunologies, and the subtle differences that make us at once similar and unique.

GOUT

A third major condition that affects the joints is gout. Named "podagra" by Hippocrates, it is usually confined to the big toe and the foot, although it sometimes spreads to other areas, especially the thumb and earlobe. But that is getting ahead of the story.

Gout is a hereditary inborn error of metabolism in which the body produces excessive uric acid, the crystals of which accumulate in certain joints, causing intense pain. Uric acid is a by-product of the metabolism of the chemical components of the genetic material. The food materials that predispose to uric acid are organ meats such as kidney, liver, spleen, brains; fish roe; whole fish such as sardines; and beverages such as wine and beer. This is relevant to its history.

Gout appears to have originated with the Semites and is recognized in the Old Testament. Wine drinking was forbidden, and all the sons of Aaron were exposed to a ritual that placed the blood of the sacrificial ram on the big toe, the thumb, and the earlobe in that order—the sites of gout attacks. I believe this ritual identifies gout as a hereditary disorder.

Archaeologists identified an Egyptian mummy that had swellings in the foot, and especially in the big toe. Analysis of the toe joint disclosed crystals of uric acid. Because gout was unknown in Egypt at the time, it wasn't surprising that the mummy was of a Syrian emigrant. This helps to verify the Old Testament ritual.

Hippocrates concluded that gout developed because phlegm and other bad humors accumulate, causing distention of the joint. Its accumulation naturally dropped to the lowest point— the big toe. He also described it as the combined outcome of a rich diet, excessive sexual activity, and sedentary life. In fact, gout comes from the Latin *gutta*, which means "a drop," referring no doubt to the phlegm and humors that Hippocrates identified—dropping to the bottom of the body.

Hippocrates correctly observed that eunuchs, premenopausal women, and prepubertal men did not get gout. He proposed that castration might be an effective cure. There is no evidence that his proposal was ever put into action.

The pain of gout is intense; in fact, in Spanish the word *gout* also means the *screws*, because it is like having a torturer put the toe in a screw clamp.

Hippocrates and his followers recognized that diet was effective in controlling gout. His school recommended a diet rich in vegetables, fruit, and fish; no red meats, no organ meat, and no alcohol. Strong attacks were treated with emetics, he thought, to remove phlegm and bad humors. Sometimes he used "white hellebore" (a very strong purgative) to bring on an attack of dysentery, which, in his words, brought certain relief.

Gout is much more frequent in overweight, sedentary people. It has historically been prevalent among the wealthy, for who else could afford the excess meat, wine, and rich food. In Roman times spa treatment began for rich people afflicted with gout, where they visited hot baths while they underwent restriction of meat, alcohol, and excesses in general. Gout was sufficiently common in second century Rome that its sufferers were exempted from paying taxes.

The search for a cure in the sixth century led to the discovery of colchicum, but it was forgotten and rediscovered again in the eighteenth century. Colchicum produces colchicine, which prevents the accumulation of uric acid crystals and is an effective deterrent of attacks.

By the eighteenth century, the medical world understood gout more fully. It was characterized as a man's disease, especially fat, robust men who had large heads and coarse skin. Attacks could be precipitated by stress, heavy drinking, and rich food. Conversely, in the same people attacks could be precipitated by the deprivation of food. Colchicine aided the search for the cause of gout, and in 1848 an English physician, Alfred Garrod, developed a test for the urine, which identified people afflicted with gout.

As metabolic biochemistry emerged in the nineteenth and twentieth centuries, drugs were developed that reduce the production of uric acid and dissolve its crystals. Uric acid accumulation can now be stopped at its source, and if gout victims are willing to apply some dietary modifications, they can lead a life generally free of gout attacks. In short, we know today that gout is an inherited inborn error of metabolism, which can be controlled by diet and medication.

Hippocrates was correct in his observations; gout has not changed—our understanding of it has grown. Overweight and poor dietary habits bring on attacks of gout; they are not the result of gout.

ANKYLOSING SPONDYLITIS: "HOMAGE TO A STIFF MAN"

When the vertebrate of the spine grow together—fuse—the back becomes stiff. For centuries this condition, ankylosing spondylitis, has been confused with osteoarthritis. However, it is a distinct disease and has its own etiology. But, similar to osteoarthritis, rheumatoid arthritis, and gout, it has probably always been present, if only to a minor extent.

Nefermaat, an Egyptian who lived in 2940 B.C., had a clear

case of spondylitis. His spine was essentially a solid block of bone from just below his neck to his rectum. His remains prove that it has existed for over 5,000 years.

In 1691, physicians described a man whose thoracic verte- brae, adjacent ribs, all the lower vertebrae (which are nor- mally separate and distinct), were all joined. Such a man could not bend, stretch, or even breathe deeply—he would truly have been a "stiff man."

Ankylosing spondylitis is distinct from osteoarthritis. During World War II, when men were more routinely x-rayed, it was recognized that spondylitis is more prevalent than had been previously thought. It appears, however, that the "stiff" men with extensive bone fusion are exceptions. In most cases it affects men before age 30, and is usually self-limiting to the lower vertebrae of the spine.

Some scientists believe that it is an infectious disease with a hereditary tendency. The evidence for this is that men are affected by a ratio of 10 to 1, and scientists have identified a tissue type in men who are more prone to getting ankylosing spondylitis. It means that if a man's tissue type corresponds, he has a better chance of getting it than someone with another tissue type.

SYSTEMIC LUPUS ERYTHEMATOSUS

Lupus as it is commonly called is an inflammatory disease of the connective tissue. It can affect the skin, vital organs, and the joints. It is an autoimmune disease because, similar to rheumatoid arthritis, the immune system produces antibodies that attack the tissues. It accounts for the early observations by the Indian physician, Caraka, that arthritis could spread to the organs.

Eight to ten women get lupus for every man. Although lupus usually affects the major organs, it often results in an attack on the synovial membranes of the joints, producing similar, but not as severe, rheumatoid arthritis. More confusion.

Other similarities to rheumatoid arthritis include flare-ups and remissions of the inflammatory response, which involve the prostaglandins. Similarly, the current hypothesis teaches that lupus is a virus-induced autoimmune disease. Thus we see that for some reason women are predisposed, a virus is involved, and the inflammatory system has gone awry.

PSORIATIC ARTHRITIS

As early as 1830, a connection between arthritis and psoriasis was recognized. Psoriasis is a skin disorder that produces scaly patches—usually red—on the scalp, elbows, knees, and neck. Arthritis is directly related to the psoriasis and has been given the name psoriatic arthritis. It also accounts for some early observations.

About 8% of people with psoriasis also show symptoms of arthritis and, like rheumatoid arthritis and lupus, it is much more common in women than men. And like these other "rheumatic" diseases, it usually appears between the ages of 20 and 30, but it can emerge at any age.

The arthritis of psoriatic arthritis usually appears in one of three forms. Most common are the fingers and toes, which can become so swollen they are called "sausage digits." Next in frequency, psoriatic arthritis affects the end joints of fingers, causes pitted fingernails, and also attacks other joints.

A third type of psoratic arthritis attacks the spine in "spondylitis," apparently remaining at the base of the spine. Symptoms of this form are the same as ankylosing spondylitis and, in some cases, it actually becomes ankylosing spondylitis. More confusion.

Heredity plays a role in psoriatic arthritis, which is somewhat similar to rheumatoid arthritis, ankylosing spondylitis, and systemic lupus erythematosus. That is, the genetic marker (a tissue type) can be identified, which identifies susceptibility, but not predictability. Thus the implication that a causative agent is necessary (a virus?) and correct circumstances, such as stress.

INFECTIOUS ARTHRITIS

In contrast to rheumatoid arthritis, infectious arthritis is not chronic; that is, it has a beginning and an end, and it is curable. Infectious arthritis often comes on suddenly because it is caused by an infection—a microorganism is involved—and prompt medical treatment is required to prevent it from spreading to other parts of the body.

Infectious arthritis usually starts as an infection in another part of the body and spreads to a joint, but the infection can also start in the joint. Once the joint is infected, the body's immune defenses spring into action and inflammation rears its ugly head.

Microorganisms that cause infectious arthritis are varied and include the organisms that cause gonorrhea, staph infections, tuberculosis, and bacteria carried by ticks and mites. German measles and hepatitis viruses as well as some fungus can cause the disease. Just about every part of the world has microorganisms that will cause infectious arthritis. Gold salts, which cured tuberculosis, were observed to help rheumatoid arthritis.

Treatment of infectious arthritis usually involves antibiotics to eliminate the infection, anti-inflammatory medication, and pain relievers as required, with rest to stop joint damage and allow the antibiotics to work.

Infectious arthritis illustrates that there are many sources of what is called "arthritis" and that the body's defenses often involve inflammation. The good news is that this form of arthritis has a beginning and an end.

JUVENILE ARTHRITIS

Hippocrates first described arthritis as rarely occurring in children. His mere mention indicates that some did exist as early as 400 B.C. Consequently, it has probably been part of the human condition for over 3,000 years, similar to rheumatoid arthritis in adults. Whether it underwent any changes in virulence or etiology will always remain obscure.

Children get rheumatoid arthritis, ankylosing spondylitis, lupus, and infectious arthritis. And the problems that apply to adults apply to children, excepting the resiliency of children. I get the impression that they recover more effectively and more frequently than adults. However, it is hard to conceive of anything more heartbreaking than a child with one of these dreaded diseases.

People often ask, "Will these dietary concepts help children?" In my opinion, they will. The dietary commitment is actually good for anyone. The only admonition is to be sure that appropriate supplementation is used to certify that the child receives the RDA for all nutrients. The base level of EPA for adults—1 gram—should be adequate for children. I recommend strongly that, in addition to supplemental EPA, a major effort be made to use food in order to create a healthy attitude toward the balanced relationship between food and health.

THE ECONOMICS OF ARTHRITIS

In 1982 the Arthritis Foundation estimated that the direct costs of arthritis were $6.2 billion. Direct costs summarize money actually spent. This would extrapolate to $8.2 billion or more in 1986. The 10 million people who have severe symptoms, including some disability will spend about 80% of the direct costs. That means each of them will spend about $700 on his or her illness.

Lost wages, peripheral care, and other indirect costs totaled about $9 billion in 1986. These costs have a tendency to be spread over society in general, and that comes to about $38 dollars for every person living in the United States.

Arthritis is the most common of all the chronic conditions, which include heart disease, high blood pressure, back trouble, hay fever, and others. It accounts for about 2.5% of all office visits to doctors each year. With about 740 million visits to doctors in 1986, that comes to 18.5 million office visits due to arthritis.

Although these numbers do not evaluate personal involvement and are not even good averages, they prove an irrefutable point. Arthritis is a chronic illness of staggering economic and social proportions.

THOUGHTS ON THE FUTURE

As the twentieth century enters its twilight years, a bright century is about to dawn. We recognize that, excepting osteoarthritis, arthritic and other inflammatory diseases are probably caused by a virus. Some people are predisposed to getting one or another of them, depending on the type of susceptibility and the virus it manifests itself as; it could be one of several diseases such as ankylosing spondylitis, rheumatoid arthritis, lupus, psoriatic arthritis, or juvenile arthritis, which is the supreme tragedy. Infectious arthritis can obviously be dealt with by means available today.

In my opinion, these diseases probably had a common origin as some researchers have suggested. Because a virus is almost certainly involved, immunization will ultimately be forthcoming. But the inflammatory response will probably remain because it is a normal response gone wrong; and every form of arthritis must deal with it.

So, I return to dietary intervention. Diet can help—it won't cure—I never said it will. But food is the foundation on which the physician must apply his or her art. The dietary commitment in this book can be your foundation as you do everything in your power to reclaim and protect your health.

APPENDIX

Additional Reading

This list is prepared for people who seek more information on nutrition in general or some aspect of this dietary commitment.

General Arthritis

Understanding Arthritis
Kushner, I. (Ed.)
Scribner's, New York, 1984

The Arthritis Foundation publishes books, booklets, and pamphlets with specific information on arthritis. Write to them at:

Arthritis Foundation
P.O. Box 19000
Atlanta, Georgia 30326

Arthritis Alternatives
Gadd I. and Gadd L.
Warner Books, New York, 1986

Are You Sure It's Arthritis?
Davidson, P.
Macmillan, New York, 1985

Exercise and Arthritis

Arthritis, Relief Beyond Drugs
Carr, R.
Barnes & Noble Books, New York, 1984

Arthritis and Drug Treatments

Journals that can be found in medical or large libraries:

"Current Concepts in the Treatment of Rheumatoid Arthritis"
Baker, D. G. and Rabinowitz, J. L.
J. Clin. Pharmacology 26, 1986, 2–21

Arthritis History

"Arthritis in Ancient Indian Literature"
Sharma, J. N., Arora, R. B.
Indian J. Med. Res. 8, 1973, 37–42

"Archaeology and Arthritis"
Karsh, R, S., McCarthy, J. D.
Arch. Int. Med. 105, 1960, 172–176

"The Antiquity of Rheumatoid Arthritis"
Short, C.
Arthritis and Rheumatism 17, 1974, 193–205

"Arthritis in Saxon and Medieval Skeletons"
Rogers, J., et al.
B. Med. J., 1981, 1668–1670

General Nutrition

Jane Brody's Nutrition Book
Brody, Jane
Avon Books, New York, 1982

Making the Vitamin Connection
Scala, James
Harper & Row, New York, 1985

Nutrition, Concepts and Controversies
Hamilton, E.M.N. and Whitney, E. N.
West Publishing Co., St. Paul, MN, 1982

Food Composition

Food Values of Portions Commonly Used
Pennington, J.A.T. and Church, H. N.
Harper & Row, New York, 1985

Books by Barbara Kraus: The following books are from various publishers. They make it convenient to find the amounts of specific components of food.

Calories and Carbohydrates
Cholesterol Composition
Dictionary of Sodium Fat and Cholesterol
Carbohydrate Guide to Brand Names and Basic Foods
Dictionary of Protein
Guide to Fiber in Food

Prostaglandins

Biological Protection with Prostaglandins, Vol. I
Cohen, M. M. (Ed.)
CRC Press, Boca Raton, FL 1985

Advances in Prostaglandin, Thromboxane and Leukotriene Research, Vol. 15
Hayaishi, O. and Yamamoto, S. (Eds.)
Raven Press, New York, 1985

This series on research began with Volume I in 1976. Volume 15 is especially relevant.

Arthritis and Diet

"Effects of Manipulation of Dietary Fatty Acids on Clinical Manifestations of Rheumatoid Arthritis"
Kremer, J. M., et al.
The Lancet, January 26, 1985, 184–187

"Placebo Controlled Blind Study of Dietary Manipulation Therapy in Rheumatoid Arthritis"
Darlington, L. G. and Ramsey, N. W.
The Lancet, February 1, 1986, 236–238

"Dietary Fish Oil Alters Leukotriene Generation and Neutrophil Function"
Nutrition Reviews 44, 1986, 137–139

Index